YOUR MAN

9/16

HOW TO DRIVE YOUR MAN WILD IN BED

TINA ROBBINS

Translated by Gladis Castillo

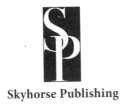

Skyhorse Publishing

Library of Congress Cataloging-in-Publication Data is available on file.

Cover design by Jane Sheppard
Cover photos by iStock and Dollar Photo

ISBN: 978-1-5107-0553-1
eBook ISBN: 978-1-5107-0558-6

Printed in the United States of America

Table of Contents

Editor's Note

In this book we look into the sex lives of men to reveal some of their deeply guarded desires and thoughts. Sexual activity tends to accurately reflect many hidden personality traits; haven't you ever wondered about someone's sexual interests?

Sex is a topic that interests a lot of people whether they are young and inexperienced and want to learn new skills or older adults who want to reignite their partner's passion. As fulfilling as your relationship may be, why not dig a little deeper and discover some of those hidden secrets?

If you are looking for a different perspective, as well as other answers, you will find more information in other books. These vary from the art of *Tantra* or the different types of sensual massage and breathing techniques to a variety of exercises, resources, and reflections related to the alchemy of desire.

This time we want to know more about men: what motivates them, what are their preferences and innermost desires.

What attitude do we adopt in order to experience erotic love after the sexual revolution?

In putting together this book, my team and I used multiple surveys, testimonies, and reports. Once summarized and grouped, it was much easier to identify the most important themes.

The final draft of the book required assistance from friends and colleagues at the Tellus Institute, whom we thank for their cooperation. We have tried to keep a friendly and casual tone in our writing, casting aside any feelings of guilt or shame that stem from certain religious beliefs or ideas about sexuality.

The following pages describe sexual practices that are not necessarily acceptable for everyone, reflecting the variety of customs and preferences in our world. The same applies, for example, with food: not everyone enjoys the same menu; what's more, some culinary preferences are desirable for some whereas for others they may be considered "taboo."

Only go as far as you want

Keep in mind: this is not a competition in any way. Nor is it a "race" to see who is more "daring" or more . . . "dirty." You set your own limits. Nobody should force or be forced to do anything that they do not want to try or do not feel like doing.

In this book you will find an array of sexual fantasies but no actual abuse, whether physical or psychological. Limits are set by each individual with the general intention of avoiding any injury to their partner (physically or mentally), although sometimes there is a very thin line between pleasure and pain and that may make it difficult to set limitations. We have also ruled out sexual practices that are commonly regarded as dangerous, such as simulated strangulation and others.

In the West, who would not feel repulsed if they were offered a plate of worms? And yet we know that in the Pacific islands insects and worms are considered delicacies. When it comes to food and sex, what some people consider a tasty treat, others find repugnant, or consider very vulgar.

Here we give you a few sexual ingredients, some old and some new, **to satiate your sexual appetite to your own liking**. Love? It will seem repetitive, obvious, and almost unnecessary to remember the wonders of love, which is not only the opposite of fear. With love everything seems to make sense: *even sex!* But we insist: *How to Drive Your Man Wild in Bed* is a book dedicated to sex.

To multiply desire . . . and better enjoy love.

Introduction:
Looking for
Something Else

Sex is the most fun you can have without laughing.
(MANHATTAN)*

What's Changed?

You turn on the television, and what do you see? Spectacular girls advertising amazing cars, attractive tanned and muscular guys offering exotic drinks . . . Television is the ideal showcase where sex is present in every ad, in every show. Even family-friendly game shows are not free of more or less explicit references.

There is nothing wrong with that; it is simply a reflection of the society in which we live. More and more each day, sexual relationships are experienced naturally and spontaneously. Women have changed their role in these situations

---

* The opening lines of chapters come from dialogue in Woody Allen films, unless otherwise noted.

and they are no longer the passive element from long ago, when men were expected to initiate any type of encounter.

Many women now work outside the home, which has given us a different perspective of life. Not staying home waiting for a man, and getting out to earn our own money, has made it easier for us to come in contact with them as equals, vying for the same positions. This not only gives us a new outlook, it also has its own consequences when it comes to intimate relationships.

The New Era

If you are in a club or an entertainment venue and spot a cute guy, you no longer have to try to get him to notice you, give you his approval, and wait for him to approach you. Now you can take the initiative without looking like an "easy girl" (which is a horrible term, right?) And yet, as we will see, all these changes have brought along other problems.

In bed we have also ceased to be passive, no longer participating solely for their pleasure without regard for our own. There was a time when a woman had to hide her orgasms because if she seemed to enjoy them then that meant that she was "a whore." Today, men know that you also have a body that responds to sexual stimuli and needs to be pleasured. Although it is not easy to break years—centuries—of male domination, we will first learn how to show them the things we like and then discover which ones they like.

It's Up to You

That is the aim of this book. Help you figure out how you can turn a nice relationship into one that satisfies you to the fullest. There are plenty of things you can be doing to make your partner lose his head and "go crazy" with pleasure. I challenge you to discover it together. Do you dare?

Some authors recommend that you never lend out your books, because generally once they leave your home, you will never see them again. I disagree, so if this book is useful to you I would like for you to pass it along to your friends, your co-workers, any woman whom you think may need it. You can also suggest that they buy it for themselves, but the main goal here is to spread the word, tell the women of the world, "Hey, wake up, let us do something to make them lose their heads over us!"

Anyway, I'll let you start reading. You do not need to wait until you are done reading the book before you start putting it into practice. You can get started on page one! Look up what you want to do most, then set your body and your mind free. And above all else, enjoy!

A Bit
of Psychology

I am devoured by my devouring fear of being devoured
by your devouring desire for me to devour you.
—R. D. LAING

First of all, start feeling uninhibited, let your hair down a little, watch your fears—we all have some fear—and, above all, do not fear ridicule. A couple makes up a unit and one partner cannot do anything for the other if he or she won't do it for themselves.

In fact, do not try using potions, magical recipes, or aphrodisiacs to transform into wild animals in bed. An intense sexual life requires something much more basic and essential: thinking of sex as a normal part of life that you can make time for at any moment.

The following tips can help you get there naturally.

The Body, Spirit, and Lust

Human beings are at the bottom rung in animal evolution. What sets us apart is that we have a **soul**, which can be a problem because oftentimes misunderstood spirituality can be hindering. Have you ever gone to a zoo? Or maybe you are lucky enough to live surrounded by nature. Animals frolic stress free, oblivious to everything, and enjoying themselves, nothing more.

Is the enemy of spirituality lust? Of course not. You just need to read about crazy mystical love to see how important it is not to confuse things. Everything has its place, whether it is taboos or social conventions. Contrary to what organized religions teach, you can be perfectly mystical and also "horny." Now that no one can hear us, we could say that one is almost essential for the other.

Throughout history, male erotic impulses have been controlled by morality. Women were not treated any better. It was thought that the only purpose for sex was to have children; pleasure was to be denied and, in some cases, seeking pleasure resulted in brutal physical punishment.

Decades ago we spoke of women's liberation; now it is time for another revolution, the liberation of values for both male and female sexuality. It is about finding sexual balance.

A look in the mirror. I was once asked if it was possible to have satisfying and fulfilling sex without having a beautiful and shapely body. This is the first notion we need to get past! Forget about your body: to respect yourself, lose "respect" for it! I'll explain a simple exercise that I strongly recommend you do before you continue reading.

Stand in front of a full-length mirror. Naked. Take a good look at yourself: legs, hips, breasts, belly. Yes, that means your ass too. Now stop for a moment and put your thumb and forefinger of each hand inside your mouth. Open your fingers as you tighten the lips until you see your teeth and gums. Now try to open and close your mouth, and if you are not laughing already, keep looking at your reflection in the mirror. Do you feel ridiculous? Of course you do. The body is just the packaging for who we really are. Who cares about being tall, short, chubby, or having spectacular breasts? Incidentally, some of my male friends have told me they love girls with small breasts (and those with more experience have also learned to appreciate other things . . .).

The image reflected in the mirror is just that, an image, and you have to accept it with joy. So when you put on that dress you love and notice some extra rolls, remember that true beauty is underneath, and it comes from within, and that is the only thing that matters when it comes to sex. No one stops desiring someone else because they have a big butt or because they weigh a few more pounds; during sex all that is irrelevant. But a bad attitude can destroy relationships sometimes.

Letting Go

Letting go is an extremely important part of indulging in pleasurable experiences. It's a feeling you will recognize when you start to feel slightly euphoric, as if you had one too many.

If you are being too self conscious, wanting to control everything at all times, it will make it difficult for pleasure to flow.

Think of something ordinary, like a tasty plate of food. You might enjoy taking it all in for a moment, but if you stop to observe it for too long you might get sick of it and end up throwing it out the window. Or try looking at a painting.

It may seem beautiful. Stand far away until all you can see is a colorful blur. What do you think? Surely it looks terrible; and if you get too close to it, all you will see are brush strokes without any form. For you to enjoy it, you need to create some distance. The same applies to sex. You have to let go of your body and your mind and instead listen to "the voice of conscience."

Remember earlier when we talked about animals and their full freedom when mating? When it comes to sex, there is a certain feeling of intoxication that can only be experienced when you let go. What we understand as bodily reactions for animals, in humans these same responses are questioned: pheromones, estrus, and so on. But why? Why can't we have that same freedom? Or is it that we do have it but we just don't know how to use it?

Creativity and sincerity. In life, and especially with regards to sex, creativity is fundamental. No, I do not mean for you to go and make up a thousand erotic fantasies to surprise your partner, it is not just about that. It is about creating your own worldview, experiencing your own sexual pleasure, ignoring myths or theories. Develop your own inner strength and let yourself get carried away, once again by sincere desire that comes from within.

There is nothing more provocative than genuine sexual desire.

Sex is an entirely subjective aspect of human life; your sex life is yours alone without any comparisons. For a moment, put aside any notions of size, frequency, minutes, and inches . . . and just enjoy.

But what do men want? As far as "he" is concerned, there is something other than his gender that makes him different from us. It is his inability to *understand us* beyond that "mirror image" that we mentioned earlier. For instance, many men are horrified by anything that seems too familiar because it reminds them of housework and domestic duties (you know: home, children, laundry . . .) so they go looking for sophisticated and "smooth" relationships involving cumbersome lingerie, high heels, or finer clothes.

Other men find any pretext to justify their desire for change: from a simple change of mood to a way to relieve their frustrations. Also, if they are young, things seem blown out of proportion because they are inexperienced and they have impossible dreams fueled by images in marketing and advertisement.

If they are older, the situation is the same because they need an outlet for their instinct to *conquer* each day. If their dreams of control and domination are frustrated at work, they try to find rewards by means of **seduction**, which is often as attractive as power. Needless to say, that causes them to make a tremendous mess.

So, in one way or another, even today, men have a somewhat strange idea of "conquering the world." Changing that depends partly on you, and luckily you have many resources. Remember: sex grows with **fantasy** . . . and it develops with the enjoyment of the senses.

To keep charm and magic going in a relationship, you will have to maintain a balance between **mystery** and **complicity**, what is more or less familiar. The surprise factor is very important, while bearing in mind that there are no two people alike, no two identical partners, or the *same* two moments.

What do men want? Nobody knows; sometimes even they do not know it. So you will have to take into account something else that is very important: do not force anything. If it's a no go, then it's a no go. Do not devote all your energies into something useless. Sometimes both partners want to love, but it simply does not work out. Just as a famous Nobel Prize winner once said, love is "physics and chemistry." And if there is no **magic,** you'd better think again.

The world is full of eroticism. Your view of the world is the result of your upbringing, your education, the world around you, etc., and you must admit that it cannot possibly be the only version of things.

Daily life is typically a slice of human experience. The way each of us perceives it and interprets it. It is the same with sensuality. So many things happen in a minute! Have you ever been on a bus or in a store, and suddenly the colors seem more vivid, you notice air blowing on your lips, you feel sexual tension around certain people, and you imagine completely different and exciting situations? We seem to want to avoid contact with others and yet, we are very close to each other. And the tension that this situation creates is not always negative, because we live in a potentially pleasant and erotically charged world.

More selfishness, please! What follows may seem strange or contradictory to you, but in order for you to experience pleasure, you have to have a certain amount of selfishness so that you can seek out your own enjoyment much more. They say you cannot love others if you are unable to love yourself, and this is a great truth.

It's not about having your partner and you abandon other aspects of your life to focus solely on your enjoyment. However, there are many times when in trying to meet your partner's needs or give him pleasure, you only hinder your own orgasm.

I also had a very hard time with this concept, but just think that, on the one hand, pleasure is meant to be shared, and on the other, two people come together to satisfy their own desire. Is that selfishness?

Any man appreciates this type of complicity from their sexual partner, much more than having them blindly surrender. It seems incredible, right? Well, it's true.

We Also Participate

Tales about women being passive in bed are outdated. You may not know it yet, but we can also be part of the action! Giving and receiving pleasure requires a bit of physical effort. Take note:

A bit of psychology

- Men do not have to know how to interpret signals that you are enjoying it. Let him know what you like (there are many ways, which I will share with you later) and he will keep in mind those places, those caresses, and keep up a certain speed and strength to penetrate. And if he doesn't know, he will learn very quickly; do not worry.

- Move your hips up comfortably. In doing so, you will find the angle and depth of penetration that most satisfies you.

- At times you need to tighten the love muscle (look up exercises to increase your sexual potency on Chapter 2), in order to increase pleasure during intercourse.

- In a traditional position, the man ought to pace penetration by moving his pelvis, **and you can join**

him, by moving similarly in the opposite direction in a coordinated motion. So the two of you will enjoy the intoxicating feeling that I mentioned earlier.

Patience and Good Humor

They say it is because of Adam and Eve that we are imperfect and make mistakes. You should know that when it comes to sex, there will always be some imperfections. Suddenly, what worked well for a while sometimes stops working and makes us feel insecure. Then we start obsessing. We start to think that something is wrong, we spend all our energy trying to solve the riddle that caused this disaster. And really all we need to do is relax and forget it.

Most sexual problems are psychological. Fear and anxiety are two threats against our pleasure and aim to destroy it. And fear can only be overcome by forgetting it and carrying on with a good sense of humor.

There are three types of reasons for sexual mix-ups:

- **Due to illness.** This case requires consulting a specialist.

- **Purely psychological.** These stem from anxiety, fear, or insecurity that we hold on to for a long while. You may have suffered an incident once or multiple times and instead of perceiving it as something that occurred in your life, you tend to blame yourself. For men this can manifest as feelings of impotence, and women may experience it as frigidity, which then makes them think that they can never truly enjoy themselves. In these cases it is very important to get help from your partner and discuss it together; nevertheless if you find it impossible to overcome your anxieties, talk to a specialist.

■ **Circumstantial.** These only occur once, sporadically. Sometimes we want to have sex, but the body does not respond, and sometimes we get aroused without meaning to; mental activity and physiological responses sometimes do not match.

To avoid anxiety from this type of situation, as a partner you must be prepared. So that when hand, mouth, or other type of stimulation are not enough to solve erection problems, it is better for you to go out for a drink or go to sleep and leave sex for the next day, when anxiety or fatigue have abated.

What I just said also goes for you. When, in spite of wanting to make love, you do not experience physical signs of arousal, it is better to leave it. Apologize and suggest another type of activity: non-penetrative sex games can be fun, especially if he does not obsess over penetration, as most men tend to do. Never make love without pleasure just to get it out of the way. You should not force your body; if it says "no!"—obey. Surely, your partner will understand better than you think.

Physiological Keys

—Let's do it some strange way you've always wanted to do, but nobody would do with you.
—I'm shocked. What kind of talk is that from a kid your age? I'll get my scuba-diving equipment and really show you . . .

(MANHATTAN)

Before we dive deeply into the purpose of this book, let us review some points. The first thing we need to do is get to know the female and male genital area well, only then can we get the most out of each.

I also suggest you practice a few exercises shown in this section. Not only will they help you sustain a minimum fitness level, but they can also improve some parts of your body, such as the breasts. Can you imagine getting to the crucial moment and having to say, "Stop, honey, I got a cramp"? This is a nightmare for many women, so let's try to avoid it.

There is a bit more technicality regarding the genital anatomy, but do not fret, you don't need to know it all in fine detail.

Female Genital Anatomy

The female genital tract can be divided into two parts: an internal one, and an external one which can be seen.

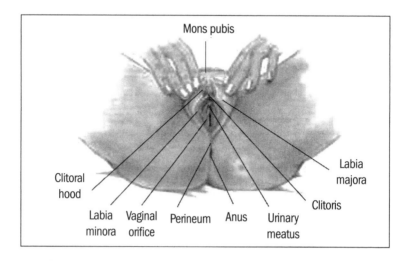

External female genitalia or vulva. They consist of the mons pubis, labia, clitoris, urethral opening, vaginal opening, and perineum.

- **Mons pubis.** It is located between the abdomen and labia, it is covered with pubic hair, and it consists of adipose tissue. Its function is to protect the pubic bone.

- **Labia majora.** These are the two outermost labia, which start at the mons pubis and end at the perineum, surrounding the vaginal opening. They consist of adipose tissue and they are covered with pubic hair.

- **Labia minora.** They are thinner and more sensitive than the previous ones and they start at the mons pubis and end at the perineum, inside the labia majora. They surround the urethral and vaginal opening to prevent infections, and protect the clitoris. During sexual arousal, they contract and open to facilitate the entry of the penis into the vagina.

- **Clitoris.** The only visible portion of the clitoris is its glans, which is where the two labia minora meet and it is covered by a fleshy hood. The clitoris consists of an erectile spongy tissue that fills with blood during arousal and acquires consistency; under these circumstances the hood covering it shrinks slightly so that friction during sex is more intense. The clitoris is a highly sensitive organ, so direct contact is not essential for stimulation.

- **Urethral opening.** It is located between the clitoris and the vaginal opening and its function is to release urine from the bladder.

- **Vaginal opening.** Clearly visible between the two labia minora, during sexual arousal it secretes a viscous fluid that is clear or white depending on the time of month. When the woman is a virgin, it is partly covered by a veil of skin called the hymen. This opening, in addition to facilitating insertion of the penis during intercourse, allows blood to flow during menstruation, and childbirth after pregnancy.

- **Perineum.** Stretch of skin between the vagina and anus. Like the clitoris, it is stimulated by pressure.

Female internal genitalia

- **Vagina.** Tubular cavity measuring about 4 inches long with elastic, grooved walls that are covered with a mucous membrane. During sexual arousal, the vagina expands transversely and longitudinally (the cervix and fornix stretch upward) to fit the penis and the walls are permeated with a lubricating fluid secreted by the Bartholin glands, which serves to facilitate movement of the penis into the vagina. The striated skin of the vaginal walls and pre-orgasmic contractions stimulate the male genitalia. There is an area of the vagina known for its great erotic sensitivity: the G-spot. The existence of this spot has not yet been scientifically proven, but try to find it with your partner. It seems to be in the front wall of the vagina, behind the bladder, and you can locate it by inserting your index and middle finger up to the second phalanx; pressing against it produces intense pleasure.

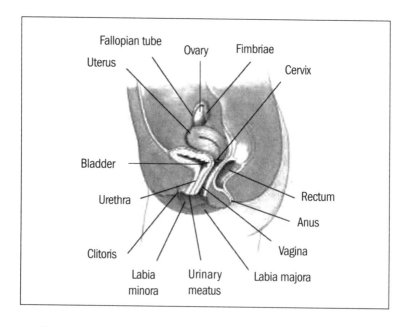

- **Fornix and uterus.** The fornix is the top of the vagina that stretches upward during sexual arousal to accommodate the penis. The uterus is an inverted pear-shaped organ attached to the top of the vagina through the cervix and leaning forward on the bladder. It consists of two parts: the neck of the uterus, the bottom part that is narrower and attached to the vagina, and the body of the uterus, which is the upper larger part including the fallopian tubes. The womb lining is shed and regenerated periodically when the eggs are not fertilized, following cycles of between 26 and 30 days (we call it "menstruation" or "period" and this is when mucous and blood flow through the vagina and out of our body); if there is fertilization, it attaches itself to the walls of the uterus, where it grows. The uterus has a reproductive function, but this is not its only task, as it also gives us pleasure: during an orgasm, vibrations occur in the uterus and some visceral feelings can be felt inside.

- **Fallopian tubes.** There are two and they stem in opposite directions at the top of the uterus. They connect the ovaries to the uterus and allow eggs detached during ovulation (which occurs about fourteen days before menstruation) to move into the uterus.

- **Ovaries.** These are two glands located at the end of the fallopian tubes, which produce eggs (female sex cells that can be fertilized by sperm and create new life) and hormones (substances that regulate sexual and overall bodily function).

- **Love muscle.** This name is used to refer to all the muscles of the clitoris, urethra, vagina, and anus. It is involved in urination and defecation, as well as sexual arousal and orgasm. Its activity is involuntary, but it can be operated voluntarily. To locate it, do the following: when you're urinating try to suddenly interrupt your stream; the muscle you have to contract is the **love muscle**. For the purposes of our book, this love muscle is very important.

Male Genital Anatomy

Men also have outer and an inner parts.

Male external genitalia

■ **Penis.** The male organ is erectile, made of spongy tissue, and covered with skin. The tip or glans is thicker and more sensitive, and it is covered by a fleshy hood, which is the foreskin. The head is a fold that connects the glans to the shaft of the penis and it is also extremely sensitive. During sexual arousal, its tissues are flooded with blood, the penis becomes erect, it hardens, lengthens, and thickens, and the foreskin is pulled back, leaving the glans completely uncovered.

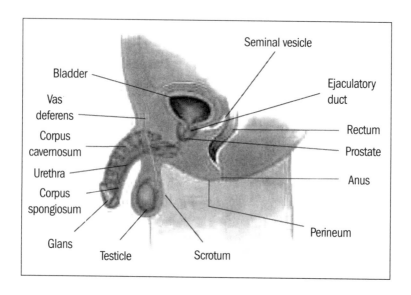

■ **Urethral opening.** The urethra passes through the inside of the penis and ends at the tip of the glans.

■ **Scrotum.** Fleshy pouch that holds and protects the testicles. During sexual arousal, or when it is very cold, it contracts and brings in the testicles against the body. The scrotum is very sensitive to the touch.

Internal male genitalia

■ **Testicles.** These are glands that produce sperm (male sex cells) and hormones. They are located in the scrotum, i.e., outside the body, because they need to maintain a lower temperature than the rest of the body in order to function properly.

■ **Epididymis.** Organs located next to the testicles that collect sperm produced in them and keep them inside until they have matured.

■ **Seminal vesicles.** They produce a fluid that provides protection and mobility to sperm once they leave the body after ejaculation.

■ **Prostate.** It is the gland next to the bladder, connecting the urethra; it produces seminal fluid (white and viscous liquid which, combined with sperm and secretion from the seminal vesicles, makes up semen). You can give sexual pleasure to your partner by stimulating his prostate: pressing on the anterior wall of the rectum.

■ **Cowper glands.** They produce a secretion prior to ejaculation that helps lubricate the glans.

How to Tell If You Are Aroused

There is a very clear sign that shows how your body begins to get aroused, feeling physical desire for the other person.

But we cannot see it for ourselves. It is a twinkle in the eye. This is often the starting gun. From there you can feel your nipples harden until the aureola surrounding the nipple swells and retracts; your breasts increase a little in size; your skin reddens, especially on the face, buttocks, and belly; the skin of the labia minora and clitoris darkens . . . but every woman has a different way of externally showing her excitement, so if you do not recognize any of these signs, do not be alarmed. For sure, you will experience one of the following:

■ **Vaginal lubrication:** Fluid similar to that of an egg white is produced inside the vagina; it slides along the walls and then is secreted. This fluid facilitates penetration and thrusting motions.

■ **Erection of the clitoris:** Blood fills the tissue of the clitoris and hardens it.

■ **The front walls of the vagina** dilate and the back walls swell to fit the penis and withstand penetration without pain.

■ **The labia** retract to facilitate penetration.

■ **Increased** heart rate and blood pressure.

How to Tell If He Is Ready

Due to their anatomy, men cannot help but show us that they are evidently aroused. You know that, right? The penis gets erect, hard, and firm. They cannot help it! But do you know how that happens? The spongy tissue fills with blood and the penis becomes harder, longer, and thicker, it comes up between 90 and 130 degrees from the vertical, and it usually leans to one side. The foreskin retracts behind the tip, leaving the glans exposed.

But there are other reactions in his body that show his state of arousal:

- **Contraction of the skin of the scrotum,** the testicles retract against the body and there is a slight increase in the size of the testicles. When an erection is sustained for a long time without ejaculating, it can cause them pain.

- **Increased** heart rate, breathing, and blood pressure.

- **Redness** of the skin.

- **Darkening** of the skin of the penis and scrotum.

- **Discharging** a lubricating fluid which can contain sperm; if pregnancy is not wanted, you must use condoms at the beginning of the sexual act.

- **Erection** of the nipples.

And, of course, the unmistakable twinkle in his eyes when you look at him, with his body ready to explode with desire.

Female Orgasm

If you expect me to describe an orgasm, I'm sorry to disappoint you. Each of us can only speak from her personal experience. Much has been written on the subject to the point that it has become a myth, so much so that for some women having one becomes an obsession, and they forget that what really matters is enjoyment and experiencing pleasure. Some women report that their orgasms are like a roller coaster ride: rising and falling sensations. For others it is like climbing on to a slide, getting to the top, and sliding down. And there is a group of women who say they have not experienced one in their entire life.

Remember what I said at the beginning: what matters is that you relax and have sex naturally. If you turn every experience into a search for the perfect orgasm, it may become like trying to find the fountain of eternal youth: an impossible mission. In fact, every moment is different even though your partner continues to be the same person. You cannot try to recreate the feelings you had on a particular occasion. You have to learn to enjoy each moment for its uniqueness. Only then will you get to reach the heights of pleasure, with or without an orgasm.

Physically, an orgasm is produced by clitoral stimulation and it consists of a series of short, rhythmic, involuntary contractions, the love muscle (muscles of the vagina, urethra, anus), and the uterus. Psychologically, it is extremely pleasurable.

When an orgasm is brought on by direct stimulation of the clitoris (using your fingers, rubbing against the glans of the man, under running water, etc.) it is more acute; many women feel a strong need to be penetrated vaginally after experiencing this type of orgasm.

When it results from vaginal intercourse, the clitoris is indirectly stimulated:

■ Vigorous penetration preceding an orgasm stimulates the G-spot, which has a reflex similar to the clitoral area.

■ These vigorous thrusts push the clitoris from within.

■ When sexual partners have face-to-face penetration, the penis and the mons pubis of the man rub against the clitoris, whereas if the man enters from behind, these same areas rub the perineum of the woman, which is located between the vaginal opening and the anus.

■ Thrusting the penis in and out of the vagina slightly stretches the labia minora, so that the hood covering the clitoris, which is simply the union of these labia, move rhythmically about it.

Multiple orgasms. Surely you've heard conversations about the ability of women to have multiple orgasms, that is, enjoy several orgasms without stopping. Sometimes it is difficult to mark the point where one orgasm ends and another begins, as though they were a single, intense, and prolonged orgasm.

True, there are women who are able to reach the height of pleasure several times in a single encounter. But do not obsess over this. What matters most is not the quantity but the quality. I know it sounds cliché, and actually there are women who need multiple orgasms in order to feel satisfied, but if this is not your case, would you really trade saying that you have had three orgasms in a row for a completely satisfactory relationship?

Sex is about two people, and one should not do anything that the other does not feel like doing at the time. By paying some attention, you can start to intuit what your man likes: how to caress him, the things that turn him on the most, if he wants you to whisper in his ear . . . just as he will do with you. It's actually just a matter of mutual respect.

EXERCISING THE LOVE MUSCLE
You can contract this area outwardly or inwardly. By controlling how much pressure to apply, you will be able to give pleasure to your partner during penetration.

- **Outward**: When you're urinating force out the urine, so that it comes out as a powerful stream.
- **Inward**: When you're urinating, stop suddenly; do not let out a single drop. Start and stop again until there is no urine left in your bladder. Do this often so you can master this technique.
- **Another exercise**: Contract the love muscle inwardly just as when you interrupt urination; contraction must involve the anus, the vagina, and the clitoris. Relax and contract repeatedly for one minute. Lastly, contract and hold for a full minute. You may notice the effect of these voluntary contractions by inserting a finger into the anus or vagina, or by placing it on the clitoris. You can also do this exercise with a phallic object inside the vagina so you can notice these voluntary contractions more clearly. The more you develop your love muscle, the higher your sexual potency will be.

Anyway, try to be careful when practicing these exercises. Everything should be done in moderation. Overstretching the muscles in this area can lead to suffering from urinary incontinence in the future.

Male Orgasm

Have you noticed that the male orgasm is much less mythical than our own? Jokes are made about it and it is considered less important. Have you ever wondered why? We said before that because of their anatomy, males cannot hide their arousal, which is usually a result of multiple rhythmic muscle contractions in the prostate and seminal vesicles, resulting in sperm secretions through the urethra. It is visible, external, and even if they deny it, most men are usually a bit afraid of failing to get an erection.

Man lives his sexuality outwardly while we women, with our internal sexual organs, internalize our feelings about sex and avoid making jokes about it. Note, however, that we have no trouble making jokes about breasts. Whether they are large or small, droopy or perky. They are external organs and as such we treat them with more frivolity. However, the male orgasm is psychologically equal to the female orgasm: it brings them into a state of maximum pleasure.

How to Increase Your Sexual Power

Do you keep your body in shape by exercising? Well, at least you know exercising is key. You've either joined a gym or tried jogging a couple of times a week, drinking lots of water, eating fruit . . . healthy living habits: you have to take care of yourself!

To maintain good sexual health you need to have a positive attitude about sex, do regular moderate exercise, and practice any of the exercises and massages that are explained below.

Hydrotherapy: cold showers. Take it easy. This does not mean you have to do without warm water. Once you finish showering with the usual water temperature, start increasing the amount of cold water until you can completely turn off the hot water.

For the first few days you will be unable to turn the hot water off completely, but little by little you will start making progress. But do it gradually. You can start by first wetting your hands in cold water and placing them on your neck and belly.

Then run colder water over your arms and legs and continue until you can run it all over your body. Run cold water around your breasts, circling your belly, buttocks, and thighs.

Remember to avoid doing this exercise when you are on your period and, especially, if you have just finished eating.

This is an exercise I recommend particularly in the morning, because cold water stimulates blood circulation, increases your vitality, and it only takes a minute!

When you get out of the shower you can vigorously rub your body with a towel. Cold and friction will stimulate your circulation, which results in increased vitality and, with it, increased sexual potency. You will leave the house wanting to take on the world.

Furthermore, these cold showers, along with massages, tend to reduce cellulite and prevent varicose veins.

Keep your partner fit. The recommendations for you apply equally to your partner. The difference is that he can see more clearly what happens when he contracts the love muscle: his penis moves.

The second exercise can be practiced at any time, although voluntary movements are more noticeable when his penis is erect. Either way, they are always advisable.

If your partner knows or has done this type of exercise, it will be much easier to avoid difficulties during intercourse. For example, it helps control premature ejaculation.

Take Care of Your Breasts

We said that the breasts are one body part about which women joke the most. We have many funny names for them. The two mounds on our chest are an area that men find attractive, (though let's not forget the butt, for which many have a special weakness). Whether by an instinctual promise of abundance or whatever, the fact is that the breasts exert a magnetic force on his eyes, and it is no surprise that at some point during a conversation he will lower his gaze toward them. A friend, who shall remain nameless, got an erection simply from perceiving them under clothing.

So, it is important for you to look after your breasts. Here are some exercises that will help you strengthen the pectoral muscles so your breasts stay upright and firm.

EXERCISE 1
Stand up, raise your arms forward until your hands are at shoulder height, bring your palms together and interlace your fingers (as if you were to pray). Press your palms against each other, hold for about five seconds, and relax. Repeat about sixty times.

EXERCISE 2
Place your hands on your shoulders and use your elbows to trace circles; do about sixty circles. When doing this exercise you will also notice how tension eases in your shoulder joints.

Correct posture. As you practice doing these exercises keep good posture throughout the day, otherwise your efforts will not get you very far. Your back should remain straight, with your head centered, not leaning to one side or the other. Relax your shoulders, and avoid shrugging or holding them back forcefully.

Your posture is a matter of habit and if you have bad habits for too long then it is difficult to break them, such as hunching over when you walk. If this is your case, you can go to specialized centers to practice corrective exercises. There, you can learn the correct way to sit and walk. They can also treat any back injuries.

If you watch yourself carefully, you can correct bad habits. You can follow any of these tips to keep your back straight and free of pain:

- In bed, use a thinner pillow to avoid elevating your head.

- Avoid sleeping on a very soft mattress.

- When you sit, place both feet on the floor, knees at right angles, legs uncrossed.

- Try to wear low or medium-heeled shoes, but make sure they are not completely flat.

- Do not tighten your bra straps too much; excessive tension can make you drop your shoulders and hunch over.

Bra: friend or foe? If you practice sports, especially involving running, jumping, martial arts, etc., it is extremely important that you wear a bra; sudden movements can make the breasts sag and cause tears in the muscles. You can find good sports bras wherever intimate apparel is sold and even though they are not the most attractive garments, they will support the entire area well. When your breasts are in their proper place, you will want to show them off in more enticing bras!

Day to day, bras tend to work more for aesthetic than practical reasons: they can enhance the breasts by lifting them. And do not forget that we can use them to seduce our partner, of course: a nice suggestive bra, a few open buttons on your shirt . . . I'm not going to tell you what you already know!

What bra to choose?

It is important to wear a bra that is neither too large nor too tight. Be sure to wear the correct size, know what fabric it is made of, its shape, and so on. Breasts vary greatly in size and shape, from one woman to another. None are alike. Even your left breast is different from the right one.

It is unlikely that one bra type can fit all kinds of breasts, so avoid sharing them or passing them on to your friends. Before buying a bra, find one you like. They are available in many colors, shapes, with and without underwire, with straps or strapless. Choose several different types and try them on until you find a size that best fits your breasts.

Bras are measured by cup size, not the size of the elastic band, which can be made narrower or wider using extenders sold in stores. If the bra has underwire, make sure it does not put pressure on your chest and it is better for it to fit a little loose than too small.

For bras, woven fabrics are preferable because they lift the breasts without putting tension on the elastic shoulder straps. If there is too much tension on the straps, your back will hunch over, you will not stand straight, and you will breathe poorly. It is quite something! Some women wear a bra even while they sleep, to keep their breasts in place. The truth is that this is a mistake. When you go to bed, avoid wearing tight fitting clothes that can constrict the body and block blood circulation.

Massages in the shower. When you are about to finish showering, start cooling off the water by mixing cold and hot until it is entirely cold.

Naturists try to strengthen the body's defenses and advocate a sudden transition from hot to cold water. The **body's response** is important if you bundle up immediately and then slowly start drying yourself off.

Run cold water over your breasts. Keep the jet under one breast for about ten seconds and then circle it with water for a minute (for the first few days it will be hard to stand the cold, but you will notice that your skin becomes smoother). Repeat with the other breast.

For it to be effective, the jet must be somewhat strong and direct.

You can also do this exercise with special handheld gadgets for hydrotherapy massage, which are attached to the end of the showerhead.

Soft skin. Once you get out of the shower, remember to apply body lotion to keep the skin soft and moisturized and prevent stretch marks. There are specific breast moisturizers, which not only moisturize the skin, they also tighten it, with the added bonus that they typically smell very nice.

Keep a healthy weight. Sudden weight changes, especially losing weight rapidly, can negatively affect the beauty of your breasts. Gaining weight makes your skin stretch and if you gain it too quickly, the skin does not have enough time to adjust, forming stretch marks (so it is important to apply a good moisturizer daily).

On the other hand, sudden weight loss causes the body to lose a lot of volume, resulting in sagging skin because it is not allowed enough time to catch up with the weight loss. That is why you should avoid aggressive dieting plans that promise you can lose twenty-six pounds in three days. Besides being false, they can only affect your body negatively. If you need to lose or gain weight, consult a dietitian to monitor your progress, so that your body will have time to adjust to the weight loss gradually.

Surgery. The size and shape of the breasts is a regular topic of conversation among women, and some give it more importance than others. Cultural trends make some of us obsess about having a certain breast size, but if you want to change them, that usually means you will have to go under the knife.

In the eighties there was a sense of needing to have huge breasts high up near the neck for a man to notice you; men preferred porn films where actresses had unnatural breasts, even if they saw scars. Now, "silicone fever" has gone down; an attractive girl does not need to have an excessive . . . "personality." Men like us just as we are: natural.

Of course, in mentioning surgical options we are not talking about cases where surgery is intended for health reasons, whether to avoid any type of back injury or as treatment for mental disorders.

Massages. Breasts, especially the nipples, are very receptive to stimulation. There are some theories about the relationship between the nipples and the clitoris, so that stimulating the former produces arousal in the latter.

This high level of sensitivity can be developed through touch.

- Grab your breasts underneath with both hands, lift them up then bring them down gently. Repeat several times.

- Lean your torso slightly forward and push your breasts together gently. Do it softly and sensually.

- Caress your nipples lightly. Lick your middle and index fingers and use them to touch your breasts.

- Grab your nipple between the index finger and thumb and make circular motions, as if you were screwing and unscrewing a cap.

You can practice the massages and exercises described above in front of your partner, let him watch, or you can even let him do it for you. Who knows where it will lead you!

Sexual Keys

I don't know what to do when it comes to women. In prison, I remember this psychologist asked me if I had a girl, and I said no. Then he asked me if I think sex is dirty. And I said it is, if you're doing it right . . .

(TAKE THE MONEY AND RUN)

At last! Here is what you came for. Now we will dive deep into the goal of this book—that is, to really make your man "go wild." For this, you have to always keep in mind that sex has to be fun and not serious or unpleasant. It must satisfy you both, so pay attention to the details. Notice what he likes and show him what you crave.

Sex should be enjoyable for the both of you (and sometimes more than just you two) and everything is permitted as long as it is done by mutual agreement. If he offers something you do not like, or that you do not feel like doing at that moment, you have to learn to say no. For example, some women do not like giving fellatio. If that's your case, do not do it just to satisfy his desire: tell him that you do not like it and give other suggestive and stimulating alternatives.

Your sex life often reflects other issues in your life. So do not lose sight (and mind!) of other aspects of your relationship, as needed. Here we will explain different positions, tips, and interests so that you can try and choose those that you find most exciting for both you and your partner. Remember, do not try to practice everything new all at once. It does not matter how many things you are able to do, but instead this is about you finding out what gives you so much pleasure that it drives him "wild."

I'll tell you a personal experience. Once I got the attention of an attractive, charming, and intelligent guy. It seemed like we had a great thing going . . . until we got into bed. What I hoped would be a fascinating experience became an opportunity for this guy to showcase his sexual abilities. A position here, a flip there. Also, my lack of agility made it difficult for what that poor guy wanted to do. If he had stopped for a second to pay attention, he would have noticed that I was not interested in that at all, and that maybe I did not mean for us to do the entire *Kama Sutra* from beginning to end, that all I wanted was a little pleasure, without showing off. I don't have to tell you that I turned him down the next time he asked me out, and since then I do some stretching exercises every morning . . . just in case. (Stretches are simple exercises that keep the body fit and promote health. You can find more information on stretching in a great many books on this subject.)

Techniques and variations resulting from sexual practice come from the privacy of each couple, so what I tell you here should be seen as suggestions and ideas, which you can then adapt to your own circumstances.

And above all, remember that sex is like riding a bicycle: the more you practice, the better you get at it. And you never forget!

Caressing

All known human senses are involved in sexuality. Touch is one of the main protagonists.

Rubbing bodies, hands . . . can be so sensual that simply remembering past encounters you may have had can turn you on. In fact, most relationships go through this phase. Think of when you go to a bar for a drink. Sometimes you get to meet some great guys. First there is the game of exchanging glances and then there is conversation, most of the time, which can be fun because if a man knows how to make a girl laugh he is halfway there already. And at some point during the night he touches your hand. The electricity that comes from that first interaction could light up all of New York City for a couple of minutes. Do you know that trembling sensation you get with just the touch of his skin?

In private, when you are both naked, your entire body is free to be touched, and not just with your hands. Use your imagination to turn him on. Some areas of the body are more sensitive than others. By stimulating them, you will get an adrenaline rush sending a tingling sensation to the genitals. These areas are called erogenous zones. Try to discover them!

- **Face:** Gently graze his face with your hands: eyes closed, lips slightly open, outline his nose and jaw.

- **Lips and tongue:** The best interaction occurs when both mouths meet. Open his mouth with yours and let your tongue explore. You can play with his tongue or put yours inside calmly and sweetly. Surprise him by nibbling his lower lip with your teeth. If that hurts, he'll tell you, but the contrast between soft kisses and light nibbles will surprise him and will not leave him feeling indifferent.

■ **Ears:** The lobes are a very sensitive area. Grab them with your lips and slowly run the tip of your tongue on them while you breathe deeply into his ear. Press on his earlobe using your lips or nibble on it delicately, but also with a touch of playfulness. Then use the tip of your tongue to outline the contour of his ear.

■ **The neck:** Have you paid close attention to his neck? What about the nape? To me, they are one of the sexiest areas of a man's body and we can get a lot out of them. You can play using your tongue and lips, in alternating motions. Moisture from saliva usually turns them on a lot and is fun for both. Using the tip of your tongue, start at the earlobe and go down to his shoulder. Do it when he least expects it, for instance, after fiddling with his ear for a while. You'll notice how he shudders. But do not leave him there, kiss his neck. Give him little kisses, then long ones, and now and then stick out the tip of your tongue to keep surprising your partner. He will love it!

■ **Nipples:** This is a delicate area. If you are not careful you can cause chafing that takes a few days to go away. But, of course, when you are caught up in a passionate moment it is hard to think straight. Anyway, you can playfully use your tongue to moisten them and avoid these small bruises. Move your tongue up and down over the nipple very quickly; then suck on it with your mouth. Now grab it with two fingers and pull just a little, notice if it causes pleasure. If so, go ahead.

■ **Buttocks:** In college I had a girlfriend who could spend hours looking at guys' butts. She even gave them a rating. Ah, those pants really showed off their ass! You know what I mean. And now there is a butt you can have all to yourself. Grab it forcefully and then let it go quickly. Run your nails up his butt, applying very little pressure, and do it slowly.

■ **Arms and thighs:** Basically a guy's arms are good for holding you in closely, and in bed he can use his thighs to better hold you. And you too can hug him this intensely. Caress him slowly and gently as you run your nails down his inner forearm, starting at his wrist and ending at the elbow. Caress the inside of his thighs starting at the bottom, using your fingertips or fingernails.

■ **Feet:** When we're in bed with a man we almost always forget that he also has feet, and that they can be part of our sexual games. With both hands, massage his toes and soles of his feet. This will help relieve anxiety, promote relaxation, and stimulate sexual arousal.

■ **Genitals:** There are many ways to caress and stimulate the genitals of a man. In the section devoted to masturbation we will explain it in detail.

So far we have pointed out the areas you can caress, scratch, nibble . . . There are many ways to approach your partner's body, and with the right combination you will be able to give him greater pleasure because you can count on the surprise factor. Not knowing what you will do one second to the next, he will impatiently await your next move.

■ Use your fingertips to caress him gently.

■ Use the palm of your hand to share the warmth of your body.

■ Use your nails: tickle him gently and drive him crazy.

■ Use your tongue and lips: contact becomes even more intimate. You share your warmth, your breathing, and your arousal.

■ Use your breasts: We already mentioned how men can lose their head over our breasts because they find them so attractive. Rub them down his back or his chest and watch his reaction.

If you want to do this a little more suggestively, use aromatic oils. Let him oil up your body and vice versa. It's a very good starting point.

Masturbation

The word "masturbation" is pretty awful, right? It sounds bad, like something forbidden. Some religions often threaten teenagers that they will be doomed to hell if they masturbate, some even claim that it can cause blindness. All of that is false, of course.

The Marquis de Sade considered it level 0 of sexuality, the lowest level, but also the main gateway through which we enter into the realm of sex.

The truth is that masturbation helps us learn about sexual pleasure from an early age. Curiosity, and hormones that help us develop during adolescence, also push us towards self-exploration. And it is different for us than for men.

By masturbating we discover what we like and how we like it. It can be a good introduction to sex, but it is not limited to that. If we start having sex it does not mean that we will necessarily stop masturbating (in fact, it is a way to relax and release tension). We need to know how to combine the two. For example, you can ask your partner to pleasure you by telling him how you like it, or buy a vibrator and use it together, or you can even let him watch you masturbate.

For men. We already said that touch is one of the senses most involved in sexual relationships, and the touch of your hand on his genitals will set him off right away. They usually like for a woman to touch their genitals. For many people, this is part of their fantasies. So why not help them fulfill it?

- The traditional method is to take his penis with one hand, wrap your fingers around it, and move your hand up and down, applying more pressure when you bring it downward so as to drag down the foreskin, the skin over the glans, and thus leave it exposed. To give him more satisfaction, try to maintain a rhythmic and rapid movement and apply pressure evenly. You can vary the speed and pressure to increase pleasure, and even switch hands if you get tired, but do not stop or you risk having him lose his erection.

- At the same time, you can place your other hand on his testicles and play with them, so you stimulate the whole area, and watch how he likes this even more.

- Place his penis between your hands and rub them together, moving them from top to bottom.

- Surround his penis with one hand, push the skin down leaving the glans exposed. Then, using your fingertips, touch the whole area. Do not be startled when he howls with pleasure.

- With one hand, grab the base of his penis. With the other hand, make a loop using your thumb and forefinger. Move this loop up and down his penis.

■ Place his penis on his stomach and rub it with the bottom of your palm. In this position you stimulate it from a different angle and you will notice how he hardens even more.

The mythical fellatio. This is one of those things that most men dream about. It requires that you place his penis in your mouth, and the truth is that although it drives most men wild, many women dislike it, especially for fear of swallowing semen—which is completely harmless, regardless of what its taste may be.

We already stated that everything is permitted when it comes to sex, as long it is what both partners want to do. Never do anything against the will of the other, so if your partner asks you for oral sex and you dislike it, you better tell him honestly and try doing something else. But if you want to try it, then this is where we tell you how you can get good at it.

I had a girlfriend whose partner could get turned on simply by carefully watching her mouth. One day I asked her to tell me her secret, because I had never seen anything like it, and she told me that he loved how she gave him head, and he enjoyed it so much that just by looking at her, he could imagine her in that position and that turned him on so much. Maybe your partner is that kind of man. Why not find out?

■ Place his penis in your mouth and move your head forward and back, pressing your lips around the penis to exert more pressure and move the skin, as if you were sucking. Vary the speed, as your partner guides you.

■ Using the tip of your tongue, lick around the glans while holding his penis with your hand and moving it up and down.

- Move your tongue very quickly from side to side and then up and down, maintaining contact with the glans.

- Lick the scrotum and go up the shaft to the glans; lick in a circular motion along the bottom of the glans, and then move your head up and down, pursing your lips, as in the first method.

- You can breathe in as you suck and then blow on it; when he feels your warm breath, he will not want to contain himself any longer.

What about the rest of his body? Hey, you do not just have hands and a mouth! What about your breasts, your buttocks, and thighs? Did we not tell you that they love them? Well, now put them to use for his enjoyment.

Using your breasts

Many women do not like touching their breasts. They even find it annoying. Well, it's all a matter of preference—and patience. Anyway, if things get complicated, it is advisable that you consult with a specialist about your breasts and even seek the help of a good therapist.

If you dare, first think about the size of your breasts. But even if you don't have large breasts, you can still do this. If you have a large bosom, you can place his penis between your breasts, squeeze them together, pushing with your hands. Move them up and down, or stay still and let him be the one who moves, or you can both move rhythmically. If your breasts are small, with one hand push his penis against one of your breasts, and with the other hand, squeeze your breast against his penis. You can run the tip of his penis over your breasts, placing them on your nipples for a little bit. If the nipple is erect, you can also try to put it into the urethral opening of the penis.

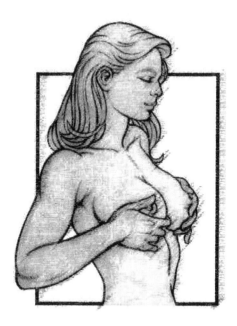

Using your thighs or buttocks

Those little sensations that can be enjoyed at any age and are almost always fun to do.

■ **Using your thighs:** Lie face down and have your partner put his penis between your thighs. Squeeze them together, try to press against his penis. Now he will need to move, as though he were penetrating you. Slowly and surely he will start moving up until he gets close to your labia and clitoris.

■ **Using your buttocks:** Lie face down and let your partner put his penis between your butt cheeks, without penetrating the anus. For more intense friction, he can squeeze your butt cheeks together as you spread your legs apart and squeeze your buttocks against each other.

Other

Touch your partner using any part of your body. The back of your joints is very suitable because they allow you to apply pressure; to do this you can use your elbows, knees, groin, etc. Take advantage of the sensuality of certain body parts like hair: while using your hands, drag your hair gently over his genitals. Use your imagination! For example, turn him on while you're still dressed and continue touching each other without taking off your clothes. It can add much more excitement to the situation.

Pleasuring yourself. Put aside any taboos regarding female masturbation. Think of it simply as a way to pleasure yourself, and you can bring it into sexual encounters with your partner, either by doing it yourself or by telling him what you want.

If you are the type of woman who can easily have multiple orgasms, the first thing I must say is congratulations! The second is that masturbation will be great for you both. For him, because it will make him happy to give you the satisfaction you need, and for you, because you will be able to feel completely satisfied.

Hands on

In principle, there are two areas that can be stimulated during masturbation: the vagina and clitoris. But your body needs to be regarded as a whole, and there are other parts that can be caressed for even more intense sensations, like the breasts or anus. There is neither a special technique nor a right way to do it. You will have to discover what works for you through practice. Find out what you like best and how you prefer it. Even one thing that may seem silly: Are you left-handed? Think about it.

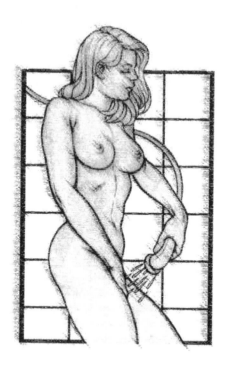

Right-handed people tend to use mostly the right hand, while the left-handed use the left one. Anyway, let's get into some of the common methods.

- **Your friend, the clitoris:** The clitoris is that area of your body that, when stimulated the right way, can give you great and intense pleasure. Think of it as a friend that you should care for because it gives you the very best of itself. To cheer up your friend, lie face up or sit with your legs slightly apart, and using your index finger gently rub both sides of the clitoris. To reach an orgasm you have to find the most adequate amount of pressure, speed, and rhythm. If your partner is giving you a hand, help him by moving your pelvis.

There are countless variations when it comes to clitoral masturbation. You can rub it up and down or sideways, lifting it up or without lifting, fast and contracting the love muscle to speed up an orgasm, or gently without spreading your legs too much in order to intensify sensations. Try to keep your clitoris lubricated either by drawing out your vaginal fluids using your fingers or by covering your fingers with saliva.

- **The vagina:** Remember how in a previous chapter we discussed the topic of arousal? We said that an unmistakable sign that you are turned on are your vaginal fluids. When you feel that this area is lubricated enough, insert a phallic object. You can use one or more fingers, a dildo, a vibrator . . . and move rhythmically up and down, using the tip of the object to apply the most pressure near the bladder area. This pressure can make you feel an urge to go to the toilet. Just remember that you are allowed to let go and release a few drops of urine. Some men love it, especially if you go on them. Have you heard of *golden showers*? Well, this is it. If both of you are okay with it then it can be very provocative and kinky. These are the two most common ways to masturbate, but do not feel limited by them: let your imagination flow freely and improvise; find new ways for pleasure.

- **Insert** two or three fingers of your right hand into the vagina and rhythmically rub the clitoris with your left index finger; begin with a deep, slow friction and increase speed as you lessen the pressure. If you rest your fingers inside the vagina you will notice orgasmic contractions.

- **Place your middle finger** over your index finger and then on your clitoris. Rub from right to left, pressing with more or less intensity. You can switch between pressing and rubbing.

▪ **Grab some pubic hair** between your fingers, pull at them and let go; do this again with other bits of pubic hair. Then grab the vulva, stretch the labia and let go; start at the area nearest the vaginal opening and end at the area covering the clitoris.

▪ **Usually** one side of the clitoris is more sensitive than the other. Start by rubbing the center of the clitoris, then apply pressure to the right, stimulating the left side of your clitoris, then change direction and apply pressure to the left, stimulating the right side. Find out which side is more sensitive.

▪ **Try exploring** different sensations by masturbating with your less dominant hand. If you regularly rub your clitoris with your left hand, try using the right hand; if you use the fingers of your right hand to penetrate your vagina, try using the left ones.

▪ **Female mythology** speaks of a place inside our body that can bring us absolute pleasure. If you are able to find the famous G-spot, congratulations! Now you just have to press on it with two fingers and rub it as if it were the clitoris, using a rhythmic movement inward and outward at increasing speed.

His mouth

Just as you can pleasure him with your mouth, he can also do the same for you. This is technically called "cunnilingus." Sounds pretty ugly, right? But it is very satisfying for most women. (Although there are some who do not enjoy it and if that's your case, do not feel obligated to do it.) Now it is his turn to stimulate your genitals using his tongue and lips. He can do it until you orgasm or use it as a "warm up" that will make him enjoy penetration much more.

If neither of you have done it before, you can help guide him; there are several ways to do it, but as always, the important thing is to find which one feels good for you:

- **Gently caress** the clitoris with the tip of the tongue making a circular motion, while inserting two or three fingers into the vagina.

- **Lick** slowly along the crease formed between the labia majora and labia minora of the vulva, from the vaginal opening to the clitoris. Go down the labia majora and labia minora in the opposite side, until you get back to the vaginal opening. Insert the tongue into the vagina as deeply as possible and then take it out, repeat several times.

- **Place the tongue** on the clitoris, contract your muscles so that it has enough consistency, and move the head up and down to stimulate the clitoris.

- **Move the tongue very quickly** from right to left along the entire clitoris.

- **Close the lips** of the mouth around the clitoris and tighten and relax them. Stick out the tip of the tongue, keeping your lips tightly closed around the clitoris.

The rest of the body

It seems that when we talk about sex we only focus on the genitals, and that our hands and mouth are just tools to help us orgasm. Remember, friend, the rest of your body can also participate in sensual games and can add an exciting element to your lovemaking. Variety will almost always surprise your partner and most likely he will have fun trying new things. The mere fact that you want to take the initiative is usually in your favor. Maybe those little details will not necessarily "drive him wild" but he will certainly appreciate them. Here are some little secrets.

■ **Sit on one of your partner's thighs** facing him with your legs out on the side of his leg and move your pelvis forward and back. If you do this for a while it can become tiring for your leg muscles, so you can change the position if you both stretch and he places one of his thighs between your legs. Rub up against him.

■ **Sit on your partner's genitals** and move just as described above, without him penetrating you. If you do it with your clothes on you will both get turned on that much more.

■ **Standing,** squeeze your thighs together and rub them, stimulating the clitoris.

■ **Place** a silk scarf between your legs; grab one of its corners in front of you and another corner behind. Drag it forward and back to give yourself intense clitoral stimulation.

■ **Sit on a bidet** and make sure that the water jet is aimed at your clitoris; if you do not have a bidet or a pull-down faucet, try using the shower. Monitor the water temperature to prevent burns.

■ **If you have a clean table**, a chair, a stool . . . with rounded edges, sit on it and rub your genitals there.

Math. Take it easy, you do not need to take out a calculator and start adding, dividing, or doing complicated arithmetic problems. It might seem that something so cold and structured as numbers have no place in the realm of passion and sex. Well you're wrong. Have you heard of 69 as a sex position? It is so legendary that all men want to do it at least once, and if they have done it, they always exaggerate their experience to impress their friends. Instead, why don't you *surprise* him—and yourself, of course—and suggest you two give it a try? You will have to place yourselves upside down, that is, his head will face your genitals, and vice versa, and in this position you will pleasure each other using your mouths. You can do it lying down sideways, or one on top of the other. As with everything else, here you can improvise and switch your mouth for your breasts, and so on.

Pleasure for two

There are also other ways to pleasure each other at the same time, and settings may vary. You do not always have to be in bed. A comfortable sofa can be a good place, or a shower, as the water runs over your body . . .

■ **Share the shower:** Hot water over the genitals is very stimulating for him; let him lather your back and once you have him in the bathtub with you—go for it! Try different positions; choose the one that's most comfortable.

■ **Sit together,** with your legs spread apart, cross one leg over his thigh.

■ **Sit on him,** face away from him and let his penis come up from under your genitals. Let the water run down your clitoris and on to his penis while you rub him.

■ **In the same position** described above, let him penetrate you while the water stimulates your clitoris.

■ **From behind:** In specialized shops you will find double-headed dildos, designed for insertion in both orifices at the same time. If your partner likes anal stimulation, something like this can be very useful.

■ **Rest your backs against each other** and kneel. Using a double-headed dildo, insert one end of the dildo into each partner's anus (ladies, you have the option between your anus or vaginal opening). You will have to coordinate your movements following one of these variants:
—Simultaneous: both push against each other.
—Consecutive: when one pushes, the other remains still and relaxed. Take turns.

■ **In and out:** Once he has penetrated you, rub your clitoris with your hand. The best position to do it is when you're sitting on him, as if you were riding a horse. In this case, he can be the one to stimulate your clitoris. The feelings are so intense that they will drive you crazy, which will make him feel great pleasure. You still haven't tried it? Well, what are you waiting for!

And remember: we will not get tired of repeating that it is perfectly normal if some suggestions in this book seem exaggerated, extravagant, or if it turns out that, when you and your partner try them together, they make no sense to either of you. If you try some of these things and you do not see good results, do not worry: it can happen; there is nothing wrong with that!

Add-Ons

Isn't it the case that, when you get really dressed up to go out, you worry even more? For example, your purse has to be the same color as your shoes, the color of your jacket has to go well with your blouse, and earrings . . . Of course this does not happen every day, but there are times when you pay a lot of attention to these details. When it comes to sex, there are days when you want to bring in some add-ons to make it different, special. Some of them can help you break the routine. Anything can become sexual, it just depends on your preferences and imagination. The most commonly used are:

Dildos. The name given to this device was very badly chosen. They do not help comfort anyone who wants to get pleasure, don't you think? Perhaps it would be more appropriate to call it "orgasm inducer" because that is its purpose: to help us orgasm. Should we give it another name? Dildos are made of latex or silicone and have a phallic shape. They vary in length, thickness, hardness, and size, so find one that suits you best, though usually the small ones are used for anal stimulation and the larger ones are intended for vaginal penetration. Ah! And they are also available in different colors.

Vibrators. They are battery-powered devices with a phallic shape that vibrate to produce sexual ecstasy. The only fault I find in them is that, since they are electric, they cannot be used in the bathtub.

Some women, especially in cold countries, speak of them as if they were their best friends and joke about the fact that, unlike with a man, you do not have to put up with them after a good orgasm.

Honestly, the vibrator can be used as an add-on for masturbation or as a sexual toy during intercourse, but it is better if you don't let them become a substitute for a real man.

Cock rings. They are just that, steel or rubber rings placed around the base of the penis and scrotum to help prolong an erection. If you want to use it you have to put it on before the man gets an erection and remove it when he is no longer hard.

First insert the testicles and then the penis. During an erection, the penile tissues are filled with blood, then the base is compressed by the ring and the sexual act can be prolonged.

Be careful and do not use other objects to do this. I still remember a case that appeared in the newspaper, where a man instead of using a cock ring put an industrial bearing on his penis, and ended up in the emergency room when he could not remove it. I can only imagine the face of the doctor who had to treat him. You won't always have a ring with the right size handy so go with a simple but very, very effective option: use a rope or a tie.

Ben Wa balls. It is a discreet add-on you can use at any time without anyone knowing. They are two metal balls, one of which is solid and the other is hollow partly filled with mercury. The first is placed in the deepest part of the vagina and the other one goes right underneath it. You can walk with them inside you, so that as you walk the mercury moves, the lower ball rotates and clashes with the other; and these shocks result in vibrations inside the vagina and give you great sexual pleasure.

I have a friend who advocates the use of Ben Wa balls. She uses them as she walks down the street, rides the bus, sits at home . . . but I would advise against using them when you have an important meeting at work. If you want to experience new sensations, give them a try.

Enhancers. You see them in sex shops. These are sleeves that go on the penis, just like condoms, but with different textures, and lively and provocative shapes. They give additional anal or vaginal stimulation. Keep in mind that they are not condoms and as such they do not protect against pregnancy and sexually transmitted diseases, but they are fun to use.

Contraceptives. The most common types are "condoms" although there are also many less commonly used options. They are meant to prevent unwanted pregnancy and protect against sexually transmitted diseases. You can use them as your regular birth control method.

Many men prefer not to use them; some even lose their erection when they put it on. Their usual argument is that it keeps them from feeling, although condoms today are so thin that they can feel as much as if they were having sex without it.

On the other hand, some people feel that condoms create a barrier that prevents energy exchange that occurs during a simultaneous orgasm.

What is certain is that putting on a condom can get in the way of a heated moment; it interrupts the action by having to stop and look for it, take it out of its packaging—you know the rest.

So have it ready in advance and find a system that works for both of you so can take advantage of a spontaneously intense moment. Help him put it on, use your hands or mouth, or give him continuous stimulation by touching him. Did you know that there are flavored condoms? There are even fluorescent condoms that glow in the dark.

Lubricants. Long before Marlon Brando showed us the many uses for butter in his film *Last Tango in Paris*, this product had been widely used as a lubricant and, of course, we can find it easily in every refrigerator.

A lubricant is a substance that mimics fluid that women secrete during sexual arousal and helps the penis to easily enter the vagina or anus. Lubricants are typically used for anal sex, to facilitate male masturbation, to supplement female lubrication, for massages, etc.

If you decide to use them, instead of using oil-based lubricant like Vaseline, choose water-based lubricants such as glycerin, because oil can break down latex (in condoms, diaphragms, and other contraceptives) and leave a layer inside the vagina or anus where bacteria can easily settle.

Look in the fridge. Of course, film has become a benchmark in our lives. There is always a movie we can mention to illustrate a point. And since I am a great lover of cinema, I'll reference another movie. Who doesn't remember $9\frac{1}{2}$ *Weeks*? Well, if you have not seen it, do yourself a favor and close this book, go find it, sit back, and enjoy it! We can wait for you.

There is a scene that has now become a pop culture classic: Kim Basinger is sitting on the kitchen floor, blindfolded, and taking whatever Mikey Rourke is feeding her. It is an example of how the refrigerator can become a small treasure trove of items for your sexual games.

There are other essential food items, if you want to start exploring sexual gastronomy. Cream is one of them. Hot chocolate, milk, honey, or ice cream can be spread over the body and then licked. Also strawberries, cherries, or grapes!

A common fantasy for men involves spraying much of your body with champagne, especially the genitals, and drinking it—"drinking you" (I do not want to be rude, but as I say throughout the book, do not forget basic rules of hygiene).

Bathtubs. Don't tell me you've never imagined having a guy like George Clooney soaking in a bath ready for you. This is a typical element of sexual fantasies. I mean the bathtub, of course. It is perfect for sex or foreplay. It's fine if you have a wild imagination but men are the ones who really enjoy getting into warm water and having intercourse.

Some women are not sold on the feeling of water entering their body along with the man's penis.

But relax, do not give up yet. Why not start with foreplay in the tub and then roll naked and soaked on the carpet so you can both finish placidly exhausted?

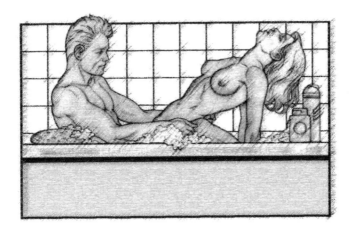

Drugs. And here I have to address the issue of drugs, a controversial issue. For example, there are people who pair up sex with cocaine use to increase their orgasm. For me this is a dangerous practice, aside from the trouble it would mean to acquire illegal substances.

I will never understand how alcohol, which is a strong addictive drug, is legal but drugs like marijuana are prohibited. Compared with poisonous and addictive nicotine in tobacco, moderate use of that plant's alkaloids results in no more than a remarkable relaxing effect, which helps some people to loosen their inhibitions and enhances perception and sensitivity.

"Designer drugs," those *colorful pills* that are so popular with teens and young adults, also help with disinhibition and greater feelings of love, but they all have very harmful side effects, especially in the nervous system.

There is also a wide range of aphrodisiacs, some of which are classified as drugs. You will find a bit more on this topic in a later chapter (see "Repair Manual"), but what I recommend and find more interesting are dietary supplements because their effects are longer lasting and healthier on the body (the book *El Dr. Comida en la Cama* gives a very thorough explanation on how to take them). Anyway, now you know my opinion: *the more natural, the better!*

Porn and erotic literature. Let's be honest, hardly anyone has watched a porn flick from beginning to end, in one sitting. Videos with sexual content are usually good stimulants for sexual relations, but not everyone enjoys explicit sex.

They differ in the scenarios, the number of people involved, how they pair up, and the positions they do.

In literature things can vary even more, although the common element in erotic books or stories is the detailed description of various sexual acts. Unlike film, here you have to use your imagination to get turned on.

In both cases, you can take note and then try to apply a few things to your own relationships.

What to Do

It is time we speak of positions. How do we position ourselves? Just a moment; before anything else, are you calm and "excitingly relaxed"? Do not worry about sweating, but stop for a second to consider whether you both feel sufficiently protected with condoms at hand to prevent any risk.

And also, as an old personal relationship author says, "Do not make love if what you want to do is something else."

Well, let's see, are you not tired of the routine? The alarm always goes off at the same time, at work you see the same old faces, you always end up going to the same places with friends. Enough! And if you feel like that, imagine how it is for your partner, at the end of the day, when he gets home.

So if your goal is to drive him crazy with pleasure, start trying something new. You know that if you become a little more active in bed, right away he will be surprised, and almost always pleasantly. Get excited and try doing something different: look for new positions for a slightly different penetration each time. This is a good way to start intensifying your and his feelings.

If you cannot think of different things right now, I will explain a few that you can try. The way that male and female genitalia rub together impacts the degree of stimulation and how long sexual intercourse lasts. For example, you can apply pressure on different areas.

At the base. To get it right, penetration should be as deep as possible, until the base of the penis is rubbing the vaginal opening. This kind of pressure accelerates stimulation in women and slows it down for men, and it is helpful if your partner tends to orgasm quickly. This position is ideal initially.

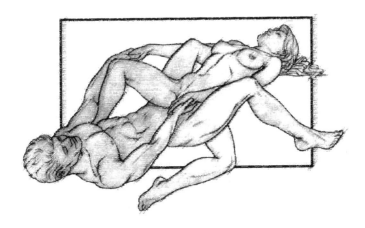

At the end. Pressure that occurs between the glans penis and the vaginal walls because of thrusting motions. Once you feel an orgasm you will need stronger thrusts.

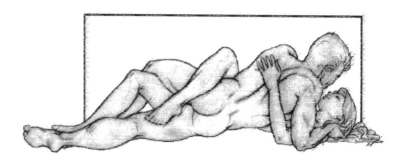

The inward movement. According to some historians, in the Middle Ages there was a practice known as "courtly love." Its main characteristic was lack of movement. The two lovers lied down naked next to each other, sexually united, with their genitals joined together, but without moving the pelvis.

How did they get pleasure? In this position the woman rhythmically contracts and relaxes the *love muscle*, pressing on the penis and thereby having great stimulation.

Then it's his turn to contract and relax his sexual *muscle*.

This type of sexual act requires a little practice, but once you manage, you both will enjoy it very much. I assure you.

One of the main factors involved in sexual relationships is *imagination*. Our mind is always spinning, so you have to make the most out of intercourse and direct that energy in the right direction. One way of stimulating it is by varying the positions.

But this is not about displaying your sexual agility and the many positions you can get into, but rather do what is mutually enjoyable and what you both agree to try. It is also better if occasionally you surprise him by making different suggestions before you showcase everything that you are capable of in one single session. He will feel an uncontrollable desire for you, but save some of your tricks for other times.

Two cultures that have contributed most to sexual variation are the Hindu and the Chinese. In the *Kama Sutra* you will find an innumerable supply of suggestions. Taoist sexual texts offer more tricks to give you even more sexual delight.

You also have the Tibetans, who have gathered their deep knowledge about inner life and subtle energies in the art of *Tantra*. Tantra and sex have much in common, but it is a practice that requires a lot of study and preparation, with a good teacher and for a long time. The results are amazing though.

There are a great many books on the topic of sex, positions, and so on. If you like variety, do not hesitate to check them out; you can try a different position every day of the year . . . for several years. The *Kama Sutra* alone offers over five hundred different positions!

Eye to eye. The traditional sexual position is that in which both partners are face to face. It is also known as "missionary position" and some sexologists agree that this position is less stimulating for the woman because it makes it more difficult for her to move her pelvis when she has to bear her partner's weight, and sometimes she cannot find an adequate angle for penetration. But you can always find variations to this position, like wrapping your legs around him or lifting your legs over his shoulders. In addition, this position encourages non-verbal communication because it lets you look into each other's eyes, and by watching your expressions you discover what feels more pleasant.

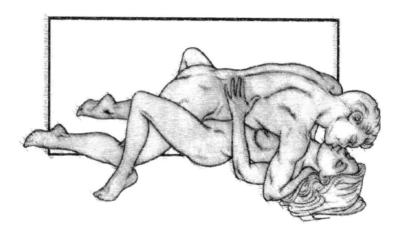

From behind. For this position, place yourself in front of him, facing away from him; then he will penetrate you from behind. To give him better access, get on all fours. Here's a little secret: once you are feeling ecstatic take his hand and have him touch your vagina. Let him play with your clitoris. You will discover completely new sensations.

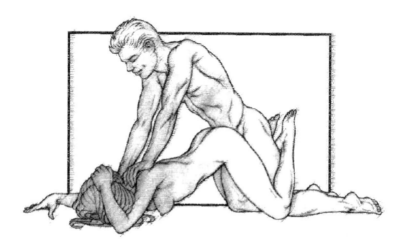

On top of him. Again we turn to the movies. Have you seen westerns where the cowboys ride bucking bulls? This position is like that but you do the riding and he . . . is the wild bull.

Once you're on top of him, sit on his genitals and insert his penis into your vagina. And you can go crazy galloping. Now you are the one in charge of the situation and can vary the pace of the movements so as to delay an orgasm and prolong the pleasure.

Each position has its advantages but you have to find out what feels most comfortable. You can also switch from one position to another in a single session. In addition, each position has multiple variations.

It is best that you discover it for yourself, but these are some suggestions.

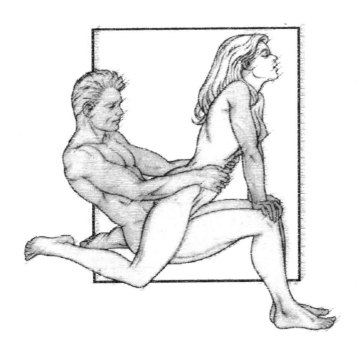

Cops and robbers. Stand facing the wall, place your hands on the wall with arms outstretched, as if you had been arrested and were about to be patted down, but in this case, the "officer" is your partner who comes from behind. As he penetrates you, he can caress your clitoris and breasts with one hand, while using the other hand for support against the wall.

The chair. Lie down next to each other sideways, with him behind you. Your bodies must fit together: he will embrace you with his arms and his hands will grab your breasts; rest your thighs on his, like you're sitting on him, and place the soles of your feet against the instep of his. In this position he can kiss your face and lick your back.

Floating. This position produces very exciting sensations because it will make you feel as though you are floating in space. He stands and keeps you hanging in the air, holding you by your back and butt while you use your hands to hang on to his neck and keep your legs around his hips.

Almost asleep. This position is great for the bedroom. Get on your knees at the foot of the bed and rest your torso on the mattress, as if you were to take a nap. He also kneels behind you and places his torso on your back. You will notice that as your level of excitement increases you will begin to move away from each other so that penetration can be faster and deeper.

On a tatami. Do you have an oriental-style bedroom with a tatami mat? Great! You may not have been able to do the previous position but you will enjoy this one. Sit at the edge and ask your partner to kneel in front of you; put your hips around his legs.

With your legs on his shoulders.
I know it may sound complicated and perhaps it will make you want to go to the gym before trying this position, but you are wrong. When he is on top of you, in missionary position, lift up your legs until your ankles come up to his shoulders. He will help you by lifting your legs. You can also put a pillow underneath your back to stay in this position.

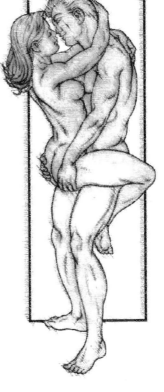

The wheelbarrow.
This is a variation of the missionary position. Once you're facing him, lying on your back, he should kneel between your legs and grab you under your thighs as he brings you closer to his hips. Once you are together, place your legs around his hips and lean back on the bed.

"Stolen."
Choose a chair with backrest and footrest. Ask your man to sit down and then sit facing him. You can better control penetration by supporting yourself with one leg on the floor and the other on the footrest of the chair.

This position is called "stolen" because in many night-clubs, girls wore long skirts and had sex on the spot without removing their clothes, just being discreet. The guys said they had "stolen" an orgasm from them. Isn't that funny?

Anal Sex

It involves inserting the penis, fingers, or phallic objects into the anus, where there are numerous nerve endings and since the rectum is narrower than the vagina, anal sex can be intensely pleasurable for both.

It is important for you to maintain strict hygiene in this area and limit the items that you use for penetration to vibrators, fruits, fingers, or penis, because there are a lot of bacteria inside the rectum and if they come into contact with the mouth or genitals they can cause infections. But do not feel hindered by this. Disinfect everything with alcohol and wash yourself with soap and water.

Initially, penetration could be difficult. The narrowness and lack of lubrication of the anus does not make it very easy. You need to stay calm, go slowly, and use plenty of

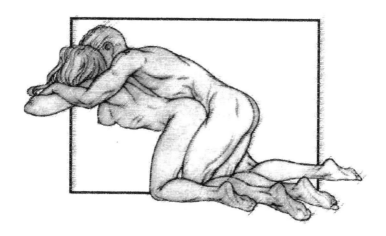

lubricant such as glycerin or butter (remember Brando!). You will probably feel some discomfort, but if you decide to keep going regardless, you will discover new forms of pleasure. Remember also how we said that your rear end is one of your body parts that drives him wild. Have you noticed that they almost always follow us with their gaze? Well, imagine what it must feel like for him to actually penetrate from behind.

First you have to prepare the anal opening by inserting a finger dipped in lubricant; when it enlarges to fit it and you start to relax and dilate, you can go ahead and insert two fingers, and finally insert the penis. Do it slowly and if you notice that suddenly you cannot continue because the discomfort is greater than the pleasure, just let it be and try it at another time. Only when the anus is dilated enough can you start with thrusting movements.

You can use anal sex in addition to other positions, such as masturbation, for example. You can insert your little finger into your partner's anus while you lick his penis, or ask him to penetrate your anus with a finger while stroking your clitoris.

Remember to clean your hands before using the same finger to touch your mouth or genitals.

Lingerie and Fetishism

You've probably noticed how your partner stares at you dumbfounded when you try on new lingerie. And it is not only because of how it makes you look but most men feel a special weakness for women's underwear.

Science defines fetishism as a sexual perversion, but do not worry if you find your partner pressing your lacy underwear against his chest or smelling your bra. In fact, this is quite natural.

Silk and satin are preferred. Soft and delicate textures are universally appealing, but as far as lingerie goes, along with bras and briefs, there are thongs, bustiers, bodysuits, stockings with garters, fishnet stockings . . .

The most common colors are usually black and red. Large department stores sometimes carry them in greens, blues, whites, especially garments made with lace. Also, if your partner is one of those who goes wild with your underwear, surprise him by wearing bras with an opening for the nipples or panties that have a central opening for easy access, for example.

It is better for you to know a bit about his taste and preferences before you "throw" yourself into this. Not all men

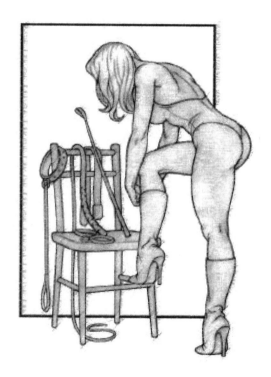

react the same to a "surprise" like this, and what for some may be highly erotic, for others may be a turn-off.

But it's worth giving it a try. One night, without any warning, you can **surprise** him like this:

- **Wear stockings with garters** and nothing else underneath! Make a romantic dinner and keep it a secret until he discovers it.

- **Buy a very sexy set.** Show it to him. Start putting it on in front of him and then invite him to take it off for you.

Apart from lingerie, there are other special objects that will get his attention.

- **Rubber garments:** made from elastic that can stretch to fit. These are items such as bras, pants, socks, and masks. Rubber allows you to define the shape of your body; that is, you're provocative, and at the same time, he cannot touch you directly—an erotically charged situation that you can take advantage of.

- **Leather objects:** undergarments, switches, whips, dog collars, among many others. You can try with a leather bra and if you notice that your partner likes the new material, then get more leather items and give him garments that you can enjoy together.

There is a long list of other items that are no less charming even if they may seem trivial. Who has not imagined a crazy night drinking champagne out of a stiletto? But there's more:

- **Boots:** denote power, and the dominant partner often uses it as a symbol in sadomasochistic relationships.

- **Black-**seamed stockings.

- **Underwear,** preferably one that has been worn.

- **Piercing:** Decorate the body with metal earrings and rings. They are usually done on the tongue, lips, nose, eyebrows, navel, genitals, and nipples. Sensitivity increases in the perforated areas.

- **Tattoos:** Decorate the skin with ink drawings. Before you do it, keep in mind that a tattoo lasts forever because getting rid of it is very costly and always leaves a scar. Temporary tattoos have become a recent fashion trend. Some disappear in a couple of years, and others in a few weeks. They are made with henna, a dye that fades away with washing. They can help you decide if you are thinking about getting a permanent tattoo, and you can also do it to surprise him by putting it on an erogenous zone, as part of your games. How about decorating your butt cheeks with strawberries? Let him discover it on his own.

Erotic Power

Surely you've heard this expression a thousand times. It defines a situation in which an individual of a certain position (political, military, social, etc.) suddenly becomes sexually attractive to many people. And this power seems to be tied to sex appeal. If we apply this concept to sex, you will find that many people only feel real pleasure when they exercise power over their partners, to the point of wielding physical pain and humiliation. They are called **sadists**.

But the reverse is also true. Some people prefer to suffer punishment and mistreatment. They are called **masochists**. They enable one another participating in **sadomasochistic** relationships.

Taking these practices to the extreme can be dangerous, but with some control, and especially if both of you agree, you can include a few of them in your sexual games. For example, you can whip each other without causing any pain. It is a game of domination, in which one finds pleasure by dominating or being dominated. You want to know more?

Tied to the bed. Ask him to lie down on his back and tie his wrists and ankles to the bedpost (the knots must be loose enough to allow for blood circulation; your partner should be comfortable so he can enjoy this sexual game without distraction). Once you have immobilized him, climb on top and kiss him while you massage his neck and shoulders using both hands. Continue down his chest to the navel; with the tip of your tongue lick on his nipples, slowly and deeply while pressing your breasts against his abdomen.

Then caress the inside of his thighs from the knee to the groin; grab his testicles and gently tighten them up as you insert his penis in your mouth. Hold firmly with your lips and press on his penis with your tongue while moving your head up and down. Stop before he ejaculates and stand facing him with your legs apart, so that he can clearly see your genitals. In this position caress your clitoris until you orgasm.

At this point, he will probably ask you to untie him. Ignore him. Go on with the game for a little while longer. Sit on him, rub his penis against your genitals and have him enter you. Move like you're riding through the Arizona desert: firm and resolute. Now you can give in to his pleas or, if you prefer, keep him tied until he reaches an orgasm.

Another option is to ask him to tie you to the bedpost and let him run loose. If you lie face down with your back to him, you he will feel more dominant and the game will intensify. Ask him to not tie you too tightly so you can move your pelvis. And now you just have to enjoy the game.

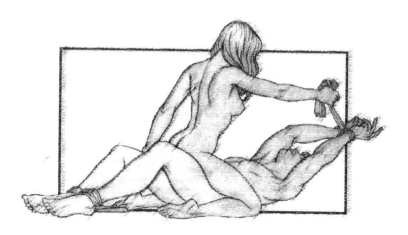

You can add another element to the game to intensify each sensation: a handkerchief. Blindfold him, or let him blindfold you . . . and wait . . .

The whip. This game consists of giving and getting lashes without any pain. When you grab a whip by the handle, then bring it up and downward to strike a blow, it sends a wave from the arm to the tip of the whip, intensifying each lash. The more you lift your arm before striking, the greater the pain. However there is a method to soften the blow and avoid injury: lift the whip up but instead of bringing it down forcefully, let the whip fall under its own weight; it will land gently on your partner's back.

There are different *whipping* instruments: strap (long, thin, flexible, usually made of leather), whip (ending in a point or a leather tab), rod (rigid and long, wood or metal), switch, cat o' nine tails (flexible leather, ending in nine strips), belt, quirt (leather strips of different thickness), shoes . . . Go in to a sex shop together and find something fun or buy one that you think you would both enjoy.

I cannot stress enough how important it is, for these practices, to have clear ideas as to the limits you want in these kind of games, because if things get complicated they will cease to be fun. If you decide to participate you will have to be very careful. Look, I had thought of naming this book *How to Turn Your Man Into a Savage*, but I gave up that idea so as to not contribute to domestic violence. And I'm just talking about the title!

Punishment. Do you remember when you were little and you got punished with a spanking? Now this game brings that into adult life with your partner. He should be sitting in a chair and you get on your knees and rest your chest on his lap. Do it while you're dressed. He has to lower your pants and hit you gently with the palm of his hand.

On horse. A very common childhood dream is owning a pony. Well, imagine that your dream just became a reality. Ask him to get on all fours. Ride him and hit his butt with the heel of your foot to make him walk. Arch forward and press your chest against his back. Move your pelvis forward and backward to rub your clitoris against his skin. When he stops, you can whip him with a small rod.

Cheeks and touches. Put his penis between the palms of your hands then stretch out your hands and slap his penis with one hand then the other. Then drag your nails up his back. Scratch his buttocks. Put his penis between your lips and nibble on his glans very gently with your incisors. Be careful not to hurt him.

The pleasure of looking. Perhaps you have occasionally surprised yourself when you saw yourself staring at someone else. Something in his expression, in his body—you couldn't keep your eyes off of him. You were only able to stop after getting caught staring. Well imagine being able to stare without the fear of getting caught. Does that give you a little bit of anxiety? The truth is that many people get an exquisite pleasure from being able to observe others. Just as others have discovered that what they really love is being watched and observed down to the smallest detail.

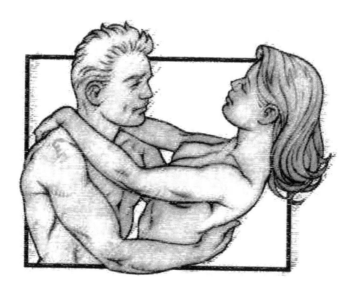

Do not be surprised. Have you not enjoyed having your partner watching you with a new set of lingerie? Or haven't you ever lost yourself looking at a couple kissing passionately on the bus, in the seat right in front of you?

We are talking about two very simple things: **voyeurism** and **exhibitionism**, and we all have a little of both. So it is very likely that any offer like this will be well-received by your partner.

Let me make a few suggestions:

- If you know that he likes porn movies, get one and find the right time to watch it.

- Forget to bring a towel with you when you go shower and once you are in there, ask your partner to bring it to you. Once he is in there with you, there is no escape. Start talking about anything, like your plans for the weekend, someone's birthday coming up . . . and ask him to sit next to the bathtub. You can take advantage of him for a bit and ask him to scrub your back. Throughout the conversation he will inevitably end up looking at your soapy body.

- Leave the door ajar while you get dressed and put on makeup in front of the mirror. If your partner likes to hide and watch, he will not let this opportunity slip away.

- If he likes to watch, masturbate in front of him.

- Ask him to masturbate in front of you (if you know he likes that).

- Ask him out to go see an erotic show. There are different levels: from a simple striptease to live sex with volunteers from the audience. Start with a "soft" show to ease into it.

So far we explored the idea of watching him or others during arousal and foreplay because looking at yourself during intercourse is quite complicated. Or at least it was, until they came up with technological inventions.

- Another use for your video camera. Place it at the foot of the bed and record your lovemaking so you can watch yourselves from outside. It's a bit weird to see yourself in these situations, but if you overcome the initial shock, you can discover a lot about the both of you.

■ Have sex in front of a mirror. If you want to watch without being watched, in sex shops you can buy a leather mask without eyeholes and place it on your partner.

Dreams, Imagination, and Fantasy

— Is sex real?
*— Even if it wasn't, it is nevertheless one of the best
fake activities in which a person can engage.*

(GOD)

*—Oh don't, Boris, please. Sex without love is an
empty experience.*
*—Yes, but as empty experiences go, it's one of the
best.*

(LOVE AND DEATH)

We said before that one of the fundamental elements in sexual relationships is imagination. Invariably, each of us fantasizes about making our dreams come true and unleashing our innermost desires.

You must have at least one idea that keeps coming back to you and at some point you would want to make it come true. From covering your body with cream and then getting devoured by a couple of big men, to spending an unforgettable night with a stunning movie star. Our fantasies reveal our unfulfilled wishes. Most of the time they are impractical, but highly stimulating.

They are like little movies we make up where we are the protagonists. Not bad, right? Too bad they cannot be nominated for the Oscars, because surely we could beat out the current best actresses.

Revealing our sexual fantasies to another person is a very intimate act, so most often we simply hold back. If you meet someone who swears they have no fantasies, you can be sure that he is lying, and he prefers not to share them with anyone, perhaps out of modesty, perhaps out of fear. All you can do is show respect.

In any case, during my workshops on the East Coast of the US, we were able to look at numerous cases of people who came voluntarily (and completely anonymous, of course) to tell their stories.

I'll explain some of them so you can get an idea. The women's testimonies start with a "W" and those of men start with an "M." Note that each story has been summarized because each case could become a book unto its own.

It is not easy to find out what is going on with your man in this regard. It is more likely that he gets frightened,

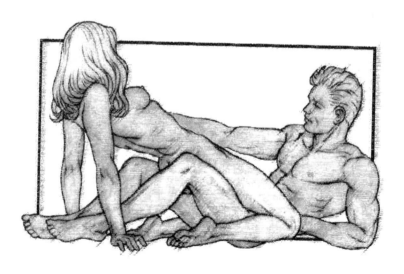

depending on what kind of dreams he has. I repeat once again: the stories that follow are just for our own interest but something may stay with you . . . you never know!

One more thing. The trial participants ranged from twenty-three to fifty-six years old.

You may see yourself in one of them, or they may sound familiar at least. Are you ready?

With More Than One Person of the Opposite Sex

W: "It was sunset. My car had broken down on the side of the road and I was hoping someone could help me. A car stopped with two young men who offered to lend me a hand. The hood was up and I was bending over to grab something when I realized that the neckline of my blouse would have let them see my bra . . . if I had been wearing one. The younger of the two came over and kissed me without saying a word. His partner came to me. I pointed to the car and the three of us walked to it. We got in and pushed back the seats and soon we were all naked. One penetrated me while the other touched me and I came several times. It was already night time when they managed to get the car going and I watched their lights get lost in the horizon."

M: "When I got home I found my wife talking intimately with her best friend, I thought I saw something odd, maybe they were being too intimate, but they did not look uncomfortable. That was also around the time I usually got home so I assumed that they were waiting for me.

"They looked at me for what seemed like hours, with lewdness, and when they got near me, they hugged me and caressed me. My briefcase fell to the ground, it opened and left a scattered disarray of countless papers. My heart was beating fast but what I felt in my crotch pushed me to continue with their games.

"In the living room, without even drawing the curtains, they pounced on me. We fell on the carpet and there they began to undress me. Her friend got on top of me and made me enter her. Everything happened so fast and that I did not really know what was going on, so I just let them do whatever they wanted. My wife put my hand on her clitoris insinuating that I play with it as she kissed me."

Being Watched

W: "My obsession is doctors, perhaps ever since I was little and played with my male cousin, so my fantasies have always been associated with doctors. This one time, I decided to participate in a *scientific* experiment designed to test the limits of female sexuality; that is, find out to what extent can a woman resist being penetrated again and again. I signed a contract where I could not back out half-way through the trial, and I could only stop if there was any serious danger to my health.

"And there I was in a completely enclosed room that was covered with fabrics in warm colors and illuminated by a red and dense light. My body was connected to a computer by sensors strategically arranged to pick up any changes in my body temperature, pulse, any spasmodic muscle contraction.

"One by one, male volunteers came in for the experiment. They only wore short robes with nothing underneath, and their faces were covered with white hoods, so I would never know their identity. Another group waited outside."

M: "I like porn and imagine that I used to be a porn actor. Before any filming, the makeup artists applied a lot of makeup on my face and body and combed my hair.

"While the technicians prepared cameras and spotlights, I warmed up by masturbating, leaning the rest of my body carelessly against the wall. Looking at my costar's ass helped, it was not bad."

Action!

M: "As I sat on the couch, I moved my pelvis up and down inside her warm body. I felt like I was going to ejaculate. I made the agreed signal and all cameras focused on my genitals; my semen shot out against them and someone laughed. After a little while we started back again."

W: "I am really just a housewife, but I dream that I have a senior executive position in a multinational company, with many meetings and so on. The meeting room was packed: we discussed an advertising campaign for a new product. The other executives gave long and monotonous descriptions of their ideas.

"When my turn came I gave my opinion: I got on the table on all fours, a deep neckline showing the top of my breasts; from my lips came intense guttural sounds that could not be deciphered, while my tongue stuck out of my mouth.

"On the table, kneeling, I started to masturbate while my colleagues looked at me without any shock. They just watched, nothing more. I went on until I had an orgasm, and then I saw how some of them hid their hands under the table . . . "

Someone of the Same Gender

We each have a Yin and Yang, a female and a male side. So it is not surprising that some of the most common fantasies involve someone of the same gender. You may have even experimented with someone of your same gender.

W: "With my girl friend, it was a relationship that took us by surprise. Her husband, just like my husband, spends more time in meetings than at home, and she felt abandoned. She confessed that to me one afternoon, and we held hands while crying over our unhappy marriages. She stroked my cheek to dry a tear, and kissed me on the mouth. I did not know what to say and she interpreted my silence as a sign of approval.

"She pressed her mouth against mine and opened my lips. Right away we took off our blouses and skirts. Bra against bra and panties against garter belt. She caressed me slowly, nibbling on my lace underwear, lowering the straps, releasing clasps. Her fingers went inside me and I could not stop moving, excitedly, asking her not to stop, to continue like this always.

"Then she undressed me completely. She took off her garter belt and we went to bed. We made love peacefully knowing that our hard-working husbands were far away."

Forcefully

Apart from homosexual fantasies, for women, a common sexual fantasy is where they have sex against their will. Actually it is an act in which she wrestles with her assailant, but the man is actually doing exactly what she likes best. Most of the protagonists of these stories are anonymous, faceless.

W: "I went out partying with a group of friends and it was early morning when I headed home, and I felt horny. Suddenly I heard footsteps behind me. I began to worry and started fantasizing. It was windy and cold. I had a couple more blocks to go and my heart was pounding. I ran, I took the key out from my purse and turned the key, trembling. When I opened the door I got a big surprise: it was my boyfriend, who wanted to know how the night had gone for my friends and me. We made love like crazy."

Size

You have heard about the required seven inches for a man. This obsession with penis size is often reflected in what the participants shared in the study. Meanwhile, men agree that the ideal measure in a woman is a 35-inch bust or larger.

An example of this obsession appears in the film *Amarcord*, by Federico Fellini. In one sequence, the teenage protagonist wants to take in his arms the shopkeeper's wife who is twice his weight and whose breasts are extremely large; they are so huge that when the lady asks him to kiss them the poor guy nearly dies by asphyxiation: his face is trapped between both breasts and he cannot breathe.

Loving Animals, Wild Beasts

Some stories that are told about the relationship between some owners and their pets go beyond imagination. There are real cases of women penetrated by dogs or animals made to lick their owner's genitals previously smeared with honey, sugar, or other sweet foods.

Zoophilia is more widespread than we tend to think, and it is also part of many people's fantasies. In the film *Poodle* by Bigas Luna (Spain, 1979), the object of desire is a small, delicate, white puppy. And now will you be able to look into your pet's eyes?

W: "Hiking at night. I left the tent to urinate and walked away from the camp. As I was squatting, a hirsute beast with stink breath rammed me from behind. I put my hands out to keep myself from falling on my face and immediately noticed how it started to penetrate me. I felt a burning sensation come over me and started screaming.

"It kept me on the ground, holding me down with its legs. It moved rapidly, giving me intense pain . . . and pleasure.

"My fellow hikers came in response to my cries for help but they could do nothing against this wild beast, they only waited until it was done and disappeared."

W: "One evening I got out of the shower, wrapped in a towel, still damp and with bare feet on the carpet. Rob, my dog, came near me and I petted him; he loves to be scratched behind the ears. He's a spoiled dog. He is always with me when I watch TV at night, lying at my feet. He likes to rest his big head on my lap while I read, and enjoys classical music as much as I do.

"That day he licked my feet and I petted him. As I leaned over him my towel slipped off. I was naked. I don't think Rob had seen me naked before. I do not know if that was what motivated me to continue letting him lick, going up my legs and thighs. I tried to push him away but I could not. He is a large dog. His wet tongue reached my crotch and he licked me. I quivered and had to hold on to the wall. I had heard of people who secretly have sex with animals, but I never thought that I . . . "

Sadomasochism

Did you ever want to have someone at your disposal, ready to please you sexually? Yeah? Some women share your fantasies. One of them confessed that listening to the song *I Wanna Be Your Dog* by *The Stooges* turned her on.

M. "He was my sex slave. I held a whip and made him walk on all fours. A collar surrounded his bruised neck day and night, and with an attached rope I tied him to the kitchen table when he was alone at home. I used him to satiate my desires and he could never refuse my requests . . . under penalty of death."

W: "That night the place was half empty, but a prey had fallen into my trap. He was a man. They all wanted to take him away, but he belonged to me. Wrapped in rope netting I got him in the car and took him home. I stretched him out on a blanket and tied his wrists and ankles to wooden stakes driven into the ground. I pinned his head and gagged him.

"When he came to, he found me standing with one leg on each side of his body. Under my short skirt he could see my vagina and he must have liked what he saw because he got hard right away.

"I bent down to kiss his body and he asked me to untie him, promising that he would satisfy me, but I knew he was lying, trying to break free so he could take over.

"Despite his pleas, I started rubbing his penis against my clitoris and inserting it with rhythmic movements, up and down, he could not help but follow.

"When I was finished with him, he was exhausted. He passed out and I left him in a secluded part of the forest. I never saw him again."

Beliefs and Religion

Arguably, one way or another, we've all been affected by some kind of religious belief, at least once. Most religions advocate **chastity**, which is typically very poorly accepted and understood. Elsewhere in this book we mention the "wild passion of love" with some deity that some famous mystics have experienced throughout history.

One of the things that many religions prohibit or frown upon, with more or less subtlety, is sex. Today we know that, among other reasons, chastity was used as a way to maintain certain "order" and social cohesion. Otherwise how can we explain that two brothers can happily share a wife in Tibet but this same situation is considered a *mortal sin* among Christians? Maybe that's why, due to its prohibitive characteristic, many people have fantasies involving religious elements (from confessionals to churches, and of course the cherished "impossible love" for a priest).

W: "I entered the church; mass had just ended and all the worshipers were leaving. I sat on one of the pews to meditate. I could not concentrate. I noticed a priest inside the confessional booth. I got close. I took advantage of how dimly lit this corner was and I began to talk. This faceless man's whispering voice and breath so close to my ear started to turn me on. I played with my clitoris under my skirt. He could not see me so he went on; as he spoke my fingers played between my legs. When he gave me penance, I came and whimpered a little with pleasure. When he got out of the confessional booth I was already reaching for the door. I did not turn around to see him."

Erotic Uniforms

A man dressed in uniform is often very sexy, don't you think? Have you tried to play with anyone in your dreams? Although there are many types of uniforms, they are not all military, for example, nurses . . .

M: "I was sick, my mind had suffered too much; they deemed it was depression, but I was actually needing love.

"I was finally admitted, after my second suicide attempt.

"The next morning, an intense blinding white light lit up my room, and the door opened; I first spotted her rubber clogs, which did not break the silence, then her soft leg, bare up to the knee. A tight uniform pressed against her flesh and when she bent down to check on me, I could see the top of her breasts.

"She gave me the affection I needed; she stroked my face with her latex covered fingers and lathered my body carefully. And then she took pity on me, taking my erect penis in her hand, she squeezed it with unusual vigor and without missing a beat she let my semen flow onto the sheets.

"She took off her gloves with a snap and she closed the door, leaving me with her scent and memory."

With the Enemy

This can be a real enemy, or someone with whom we do not get along. An example of this type of sexual fantasy is found in the film *The Night Porter* by Liliana Cavani (Italy, 1974), where the protagonist, a former Nazi concentration camp prisoner, is sexually attracted to her attacker, who after the war has managed to hide his identity working as a night porter at the hotel where she is staying.

This type of fantasy exists, although not very common, whether you agree or disagree with them. We are not sure that you would make him go wild with this type of unusual situation, either.

With Someone You Lust After

One of the activities in which the volunteers at the Georgia Institute participated, was to think "what would have happened if . . . " It's very simple. It is about reconstructing the details of a situation that for some reason makes you get particularly aroused. For example, running into your crush or a hot co-worker at a nightclub. Focus on what he said, what you answered, what happened, if you touched his hands, if your bodies came into contact, and just before you go on your separate ways, change things up and start fantasizing about what would have happened if . . .

You can change the ending as many times as you want. This exercise can stimulate your sexual imagination.

Someone of a Different Age

M: "I was sitting at a cafe in front of a theater downtown. I noticed the woman sitting at the next table and that made me want to stop by. She was older than me. We got into a conversation, and from there . . . I had never felt sheets so thin, and her body was beautiful, marked by time, but very beautiful. Her desire was strong and sincere and that turned me on even more. I caressed her legs in fancy lingerie; she was not wearing panties and I moistened my fingers inside her. I licked her nipples and suddenly she turned around and demanded that I enter her right away, I immediately did as I was told."

In the Most Unexpected Places

These fantasies bring together the desire for pleasure and the thrill that comes from the risk of getting caught. Sometimes there is exhibitionism involved and other times it is just about taking an opportunity in the most amazing places: the subway, parks, elevators, etc., are often chosen as ideal locations for erotic fantasies.

M: "That girl drove me crazy. Every time I felt her body near me, I started to feel hot sweat all over my body, and my pants always seemed like they were about to explode. We had done it in every position and place. We fooled around in the car, doorway, at the movies . . . That afternoon we were in a cocktail bar. She started kissing me. I noticed she was ready, and suddenly she put my hand on her crotch. I blocked her from view with my body as I put my hand under her skirt; I kept my eye on the waiter for fear of being discovered; she hugged me, and I played with her clitoris until she had an orgasm. We paid for the drinks and ran out, in case they had seen us."

New Technologies

Yes, girl. New technologies are also becoming part of our sex lives. At first it would seem that one is not very compatible with the other, but you would be surprised once you find out all the possibilities out there and how great they can be.

Sex hotlines, websites, chat rooms, or personal ads are just a few examples. If the arrival of the phone was a revolution, I cannot even begin to describe all the changes brought about by the Internet. Today, almost everyone has a personal computer with a view into the amazing world of relationships. The anonymity you get with a phone call or in one of the many sex chat rooms gives people the chance to lose their fear of having an erotic encounter.

Deep down, they are a reflection of the loneliness felt by a large majority of people. It is kind of a long distance relationship, which opens new possibilities for finding a mate. If a man prefers making contact only by Internet it means he is interested in experiencing new things but online it is very easy to lie or exaggerate. I'm not too thrilled by phone sex, but here are some suggestions that you could even share with your partner.

- **Call your sex buddy.** Start off with a regular topic of conversation and then steer towards what really interests you. Describe the sexy clothes you are wearing, your genitals, how you caress your clitoris. Ask him what direction his penis is pointing, if there is someone nearby, if he can masturbate during the conversation.

- **Have your partner meet you** in a sex chatroom. Both of you must log in at a certain time, with nicknames you will know beforehand, and start a conversation. This experiment can be extremely exciting because hundreds of people may be reading your erotic or kinky messages.

- **One day when you know** you'll get home late, send him links to erotic pages. When you get home, you'll probably find him still stuck at the computer. Get next to him and look at some content together and start caressing him without turning off the computer.

Expand Your Circle of . . . Sexual Friends

We have noticed that some of the most common fantasies for men and women involve having sex with **several people at once**. And why not? The important thing is that you decide if you're up for it. If you participate willingly in such *games*, you must have a very *special* attitude and mood (usually referred to as an "open" mind, but I refuse to call it that). Before taking on this kind of relationship you should really think about it, weigh any pros and cons.

Also keep in mind that if deep down you feel as though this type of thing "does not work for you," it is better to strive to be yourself, and not become someone you're not; people can experience radical transformations, but we do not have to be *someone else* and become who we are not.

Moreover, it goes without saying that if your man wants to do each and **every** tip in this book, most likely, he is a sexual *monster*.

If you both agree, trying new things does not have to be a negative thing, although you risk exposing deeply hidden feelings like jealousy, infidelity, etc.

A couple, for example, invites someone to participate in their sexual encounters and **exchange partners**. As I said, there are a couple of things that need to be considered.

The issue of loyalty is one of them. You can agree to give each other complete freedom in this regard. There are some couples who prefer to tell each other everything after having casual sex with others to turn each other on.

The other issue is jealousy. It is a feeling which you cannot fight. You could try to control it and avoid obsessing, but there it is.

So, if you're the type of faithful woman who asks your partner for the same kind of treatment that you give him, and you can get carried away by jealousy . . . it's perfectly alright to skip this chapter.

As I said, it is a dangerous game. However, if what you want is to try different experiences, and you think your man would be interested in this topic, go ahead!

Exchanges

Imagine you're in a bar with your partner and you see a guy showing some signs of interest. At first you do not dislike the man; you could almost say he is attractive and you'd take off with him to have a most memorable experience. Would you leave your partner with the woman accompanying the gentleman that you just met, while you have a great time with him? Are you sure you would not spend the whole time wondering what your partner might be doing with another girl? Would you be able to enjoy your time with this other person and not fret? If you answered "yes," then you are ready for swapping.

Cocktail bars are the best places for this kind of experience, but you can also ask around among your friends if you think this sounds like something they would be into . . . but you better be sure, otherwise you risk losing them.

One way to ensure that things turn out well: agree with your partner on some kind of signal that means refusing a swap with another couple.

Five Wonderful Tips

If she would take my heart in hand, I would give the cities of Samarkand and Bukhara.

(HAFIZ)

1. The Male Multiple Orgasm

"I realized that they can also feel different kinds of pleasure," says twenty-seven-year-old Maria. "Copying what I saw in a movie, I tied him up to the headboard of the bed using silk ribbons and I turned him on by caressing his hands and mouth until he was ready to melt like caramel. Then, instead of continuing or untying him, I paused for a few minutes and stopped touching him. I did this three times, bringing him to the brink of an orgasm each time, until he was begging, pleading with me not to stop again, and to keep going already. When I granted his wish, he had the most intense and powerful orgasm I've ever seen. He trembled from head to toe, and spent the rest of the night thanking me. It sounds trite, but the truth is that, ever since, I feel like he is my 'sex slave,' always open to anything I want."

Men are able to have several types of orgasms, much like women; orgasms can range from a subtle chill to the most maddening contractions, depending on the type of stimulation they get. We are not the only ones that are fortunate enough to experience several orgasms in a row. They have spent centuries squandering the power they embody, because they wrongly believe that there is no orgasm without ejaculation.

If a man ejaculates he needs to have a rest period, which can last from fifteen minutes to three or four hours. That is usually the time needed before getting another erection, and during which it is impossible to enjoy another orgasm immediately. That is why it is important for him to learn how to climax without releasing any semen.

Elsewhere in this book we make reference to Eastern observations on the benefits of avoiding unnecessary ejaculations to enjoy a long and vigorous life.

You need to help him get there. This means that you have to train him so that when you see that he is about to orgasm, you stop cold and help him delay it by doing one of our suggestions below. In addition, he should contract the love muscle (just like we do, as though he were interrupting his urine flow).

This trick stops sperm output, but he has to exercise those muscles beforehand by contracting and relaxing them for about ten seconds, twenty to thirty times a day. He can do this at any time, even when urinating: he just needs to stop urinating and then continue at short intervals.

After a week the results are noticeable, but it's better if he can do it for about a month. With some skill, your man will be able to stop ejaculation even during an orgasm, which guarantees that he will climax more than once. Does it sound complicated? It's all a matter of wanting it enough and having patience.

2. Secrets of the East: Massage Him from Within You

Let's try another trick. Do you want his pleasure to last and last? There are gradual arousal techniques that can keep him at that stage where he feels "I'm coming, I'm coming" for longer than you had ever imagined, which makes an orgasm that much more explosive. Asians are centuries ahead of us in terms of having refined the arts of lovemaking, whether we look at the Chinese Taoists or at the tantric postures of the *Kama Sutra*, some of which you will find elsewhere in this book.

Here we are talking about a secret that many women in the Far East have mastered. It consists of "massaging" his penis inside you by contracting the inner muscles of the vagina (pubococcygeus muscle). In the West we may see Thai jugglers throwing balls or inhaling a cigarette with their vagina: what we are suggesting has *nothing to do* with this kind of oddity, but rather it is about taking advantage, naturally, of your own body's less known capabilities.

Remember that for you to master this technique you need complete control of your vaginal muscles, for which you just have to interrupt your urine. Contract your vaginal muscles and count to ten before relaxing again. Practice twenty times a day for a couple of weeks. These are Kegel exercises that turn you into what the *Kama Sutra* calls a "gripper," that is, a girl capable of massaging the penis of her beloved from inside her vagina.

They also help increase your own pleasure and maintain, or help you recover, the firmness of the muscle wall of your vagina. Moreover, gynecologists recommend them after delivering a baby.

Try it after you have had some practice. When he's inside you, contract your vagina around his penis. You'll notice that his erection grows and becomes more intense: that is the moment when you have to contract those muscles intermittently, gradually increasing in strength and speed. Men really appreciate this ability because of how impressive their results are.

3. A Call to Eros

This is a small activity you can do during foreplay: it brings together two erogenous zones. The easiest way is to connect a body part (for instance, nipples, ears, neck, or thighs) and the penis. It is a double stimulation that brings him very high levels of pleasure.

You can start stimulating not only his penis but any other erogenous zone, for example, if he likes, his nipples. Caress his penis and at the same time kiss him on the chest, with synchronized movements going in the same direction, applying constant pressure. Then leave his chest alone and focus just on his penis and then go back to the chest, asking him to focus on his nipples. This is one way to train him so that when you get close to his nipples, he will feel a tingling reflex in his penis.

4. His G-Spot

We insist that men, just like us, can experience different types of orgasms with varying degrees of intensity. And they can even experience multiple orgasms in a single session. Do men have a G-spot? Some experts believe that they do and that it is located in the perineum, the area between the testicles and the anus. Since there are many nerve endings there, it can help unleash a very different kind of orgasm than the one obtained by exclusively stimulating the penis.

When that area is pressed (see drawing) the prostate is stimulated, a point with multiple nerve endings beneath the male bladder. By exerting gentle pressure there, using your tongue or fingers, you can make him feel different waves of pleasure compared to those obtained from only stimulating the penis.

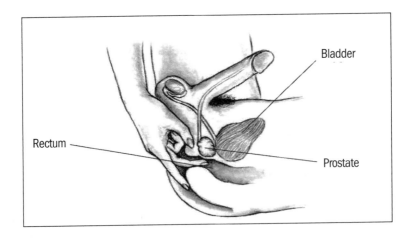

You can also stimulate the penis and perineum at the same time using your hands and mouth. As this testimony goes: "My girlfriend knows just what to do to get me going; first she stimulates my penis until I feel like I am about to lose it, and just then she starts to apply pressure on me (the perineum) with her thumb. She jerks me off with one hand and with the other hand she pushes on that part of my body, a bit like she is ringing a doorbell. After a few seconds I start to quiver from head to toe and I feel chills all over my body. I feel like a volcano that is close to erupting."

5. Last Longer with Raging Pleasure

There's nothing like turning him on, pausing, and starting again from the beginning. Get him to the point where he is about to finish and then . . . wham! Pull back. That helps you maintain a certain seduction level the entire time.

When a man is on the verge of an orgasm all his muscles tense; so if you stop stimulation at the right time, you can manage to increase his sexual tension. Then when he finally releases it, the feeling will be even greater.

See if you know (or try to discover) when he is just about ready to explode: his thighs and buttocks tighten and tremble, his breathing and heartbeat increase . . .

In that moment, compress his glans with your hands, press it between thumb and forefinger. Although you will be applying pressure it will not hurt him, but it will stop ejaculation (it is usually recommended as an exercise for those suffering from premature ejaculation), and his erection might go down slightly for a moment.

There are girls who try a different trick: gently pulling on the testicles just as he is about to finish. In this case, do it carefully, because this is a sensitive area. His scrotum shrinks and pulls in toward his body, so by pulling on them you counteract his orgasm. After you do this two or three times, he will be begging you to let him enjoy already: then it is time for you to grant him his wish . . .

Another Point of View

—Men and women want very different things out of sex. They've never forgiven each other.
—Where would you say love came in?
—There's only one kind of love that lasts—unrequited love. It stays with you forever.

(SHADOWS AND FOG)

Final Recommendations

So far this summary of activities, tips, and tricks are meant to make your partner howl with pleasure in bed. As I explained, it is not just about showcasing **everything** you learn. Remember that it is better to do just a few things but do them well. There is another important component of your relationship that you must cultivate. Attracting a man and getting him to lose his head over you also requires other kind of effort and some **extra effort**. Try to come up with other sexy things you can do for him. I started making a list, which I expanded on, or crossed out, according to the responses I got. Here are a few suggestions, with the caveat that some of them (for example, waking him up at three in the morning) cannot be entirely to his liking. The rest I leave to your imagination and intuition.

1. Wake him up early in the morning, against his pleas (on days when your offer will be well received).
2. Take some photos of yourself in the bathroom, wearing nothing but underwear, and text them to him.
3. Offer to shower together, so you can lather him.
4. Get new lingerie.
5. Do a striptease for him wearing your new lingerie.
6. Show him how you masturbate.
7. Stock up on strawberries or cherries. Place one on your chest and invite him to eat it.
8. Now put one in your vagina and ask him to do the same.
9. Leave him erotic notes where he may find them.
10. Get a hotel room and check-in as "the Smiths."
11. Provoke him sexually in public places, discreetly rubbing his privates with your hand.
12. Put your hand in his front pocket with the excuse of needing a handkerchief, a quarter, whatever . . . and instead, touch him for a few seconds.
13. Take him out for dinner and let him know that you are not wearing panties.
14. At the restaurant, take your shoes off, stretch your leg under the table and place your foot on his crotch. Massage him using your toes.
15. Share a bottle of wine and pour a little over your body for him to drink.
16. Fill a new pair of stilettos with champagne and invite him to drink.
17. Get a pair of back-seamed panty hose. Put on a tight skirt and a slightly low-cut blouse. Ask him to take you out.
18. Meet him at a cocktail bar and pretend you do not know him. Have him try to woo you again.

19. Masturbate together in the morning before going to work.
20. Buy flavored or color condoms. Fluorescent ones glow in the dark (turn off the bedroom lights).
21. Start to caress his crotch while he is on the phone with his mother or boss.
22. Try a new position from time to time.
23. Take him clothes shopping at a large department store and ask him to join you in the dressing room.
24. Give him a sensual or very sexual movie like $9\frac{1}{2}$ *Weeks*. (Or similar).
25. Ask him to let you blindfold him, and do things to him that he won't easily forget.

Are you taking notes? And what are you waiting for! Why not start today? Now? Already!

The End of Sex

The American writer and aikido master George Leonard is the author of a number of books and articles related to the body, mind, and spirit. After working for years as a magazine editor, in 1983 he wrote *The End of Sex*, a book related to the state of erotic love after the sexual revolution. We selected a few passages to help us understand the whys. Why all this? Why this collection of tricks and little secrets related to men?

Recently, a man told me about meeting someone at one of those places where hooking up seems likelier: bars, or musical venues that make it easier to meet people. A woman sat at the bar next to him and, without even saying hello, she said, "I want to be perfectly straightforward with you. Do you want to go home and fuck?" Her invitation, which he turned down this time, represents an ideological triumph for sexual liberation and female aggression. Today, phrases that once would have been considered scandalous just make us yawn. Recreational sex fails because it is boring and not because it is immoral. Their plot can be summarized, Hollywood-style, in three stages:

Guy meets girl. Guy gets the girl. They go their separate ways.

By contrast, even the most hackneyed story of "boy meets girl" has at least a hundred different possibilities. The desire for romance is a universal human characteristic. The best affairs, like the best games, are full of suspense, narrow escapes, interesting conflicts, and satisfying resolutions. From this point of view, romantic love, with longing, danger and despair, separations and reunions, is the one we identify with the most in the broadest sense. Purely recreational sex, however, detracts, turning the story into something monotonous, repetitive, and boring.

So speeches, books, and films about sexual experiments pale in comparison to truly spontaneous, deep, and erotic love. Love (is there any doubt?) is the human expression of creative energy that covers the earth with immense forests or allows for primitive marine creatures to breathe, run, or fly.

Eroticism, energy, and ecstasy. It is life-giving energy and the force that will ultimately unify the world. If we could only see it for what it truly is, every act of love would seem to us like an affirmation and continuation of life. Two people united by erotic love have the chance to create their own energy field, which is something unique in the world. It is a union that arises not necessarily for procreation, but for creation; they release new information, new energy, and a new light form somewhere into the universe.

So we can say that an erotic encounter brings us closer to a state of ecstasy. It allows each of us to take off our masks, destroy any facades we present to the world, and temporarily exist in a pure state without expectations or preconceived notions. We slowly peel off layers that we created through our physical appearance and habits. First we take off our clothes; then we get rid of all other social indicators: profession, titles, honors, bank account. Decorum disappears and with it our pride.

My freedom is based precisely on surrender and my willingness to abandon the personality I've created for myself ("persona" is a Greek word meaning "mask"), the image of who I am in the world and what I should be: my ego. If I am willing to get to this point without expecting anything from my partner, then I cannot be wrong. There are no "sexual" problems" or "sexual solutions." I am like a god, whatever happens. Thus, in this state of openness and surrender, renouncing all "effort," I can fulfill all of my erotic potential. I'm willing to lose everything and find nothing. Under these circumstances, everything we learn in the ordinary world is useless: grammar, syntax, the acuteness of the senses . . .

Erotic love is too important for us to repress it, and it is also too important for us to devalue it.

Open up to the unpredictable. Trust is the flip side of surrendering and we cannot establish a deep connection unless we surrender—without seeking ownership of the other person because the mere idea of someone "belonging" to us makes them become an object. This is about being willing to give or receive in unpredictable and mysterious ways, which does not necessarily involve what we understand as "vulgar."

In the world of quantum physics, the more we know the position of an elementary particle, the less we know about its momentum. In love, the more we try to have our lover express his opinion, the fewer feelings and impulses we experience. There should be no obligations or expectations imposed on our lover.

Danger, insecurity, and a hint of the forbidden are ingredients that increase our mutual excitement every moment we spend together.

The splendor of erotic love gives us an opportunity to engage in a passionate relationship with another human being and, through him, with the universe. Love connects us with other human beings, with everyone, and certainly even with the stars.

What Kind of Relationship Do You Want?

This question may surprise you nowadays, but if you want to experience an exquisite sexual encounter then your answer should be clear. In the *Kama Sutra*, Vatsyayana describes up to eight categories or sexual liaisons ranging from the ambiguous union, or "haystack" (satisfying a sexual impulse and no more, often with prostitutes) to love at first sight, where two lovers are truly shackled by passion.

Needless to say that when you match your partner, that is, when both of you share the same feeling, then sexual intercourse takes another dimension, and tenderness, complicity, and affection result in pleasure that gets renewed time and time again.

"I'm too old for this . . . " This book is for people of all ages. It's never too late to live the wonderful experience of love! Except in the case of illness, any fear or any excuse is just a *limitation* that keeps us from moving toward self-knowledge and self-improvement.

We reinvent ourselves every day. Depending on how we reinvent ourselves (and, especially, as we live, as we feel) we can cultivate happiness in one way or another.

Whether you want to have new experiences, strengthen a relationship, or rekindle the fire with your partner, the tricks and tips found in this book can help you adopt new ideas. You'd be amazed at the results! Now, it is up to you to decide. You choose. Do not force yourself to do anything you do not want.

You'll notice that throughout this book there are *psychological* tidbits (very simple and very few really, if you consider their importance). We have tried to be brief and practical, but we recognize the crucial role of the mind when it comes to sensual topics. Especially for men, it is said that "the brain is the first sexual organ."

Why a bit of psychology? It helps us be more self-aware and gives us perspective.

Fears. We have talked about fear. Remember that one of the first fears you need to overcome is **fear of ridicule**. That type of fear is ridiculous!

Are you afraid of comparisons? Our poor men do suffer with comparisons! When it comes to sex there could be "someone better than you," but think instead that there are certainly people who are "worse than you." Even for someone who is an expert in the arts of seduction and sex, there is no guarantee that they will feel that special "chemistry" necessary for making a relationship work.

So stay calm. And remember the wise advice of a great yogi: "An ounce of practice is worth more than tons of theory."

Goddesses and prostitutes. (What will he think of me? He'll think I'm slutty . . .)

Keep in mind that a few thousand years ago, sexuality was sacred. And when I say "sacred," I do not mean in a context of organized religion, our current understanding of morality, nor procreation, etc. We are referring to the fact that, for primitive tribes, worshipping their respective goddess meant, above all, a respect for Mother Nature and for the myths and symbols that explained the natural world better than any other theory.

So *you* are the goddess: reveal the goddess within you! Although sometimes there is a thin line between a goddess and a prostitute to the point that we might get them easily confused.

Now, do you really want to make him go wild? Well you're in luck, because your task, depending on how you put it into practice, can be a great art, which begins with yourself, your self-worth, and your **self-esteem** (remember that if this is low, you have to work on that too). In this incessant dance of energies you're going out to *dance*. This is an exciting adventure, where you will learn more about yourself.

You might think: *This is pathetic! I'll just make a fool of myself!* It could be. Even if you don't do everything we describe here, it is quite possible that at some point it may feel like that. But so what! The world will not end in one day. Some of the ideas that we offer you may seem (and could be considered) pathetic, at a given moment. But just laugh. Laugh all you can, because the whole universe will laugh with you. Other times you will enjoy a different suggestion so much that you (both) feel sublime.

Practice will help you decipher when you want and need one thing and not another. And when (and how) he perceives you during your sexual encounters. Once you know that part well, you are halfway there.

Always the same, always different. Just as there are no rules in love, when it comes to sex, there is no "norm." It may be that "normal" is amazing. Every loving union between two human beings provides a unique and different situation every time. So if you add a higher dose of creativity to your daily life you will also get better results in bed.

Your sex life is almost always a reflection of everything else in your life; if some things weigh more than others, it will be the same when it comes to sex.

For example, you may find that if you are *chatty*, you bore your partner with words (this can also happen to him, of course). The same if you feel more romantic, or rather intellectual, or given to relevant or inconsequential issues. Reactions can be as varied as unexpected.

One of the nice things about sexual activity, apart from being able to satisfy our own pleasure and the feeling of sharing energy, is precisely that point of uncertainty that pushes us toward desire until the end of our lives.

And what about tenderness? This is the title of an old French film (*Et la tendresse? . . . Bordel!*) from the New Wave era that explores the relationships of three couples. Among the three types—romantic couple, patriarchal couple, and tender couple—only the last one seemed to show lasting possibilities. The romantic couple ended with the man seeking extramarital affairs, and the patriarchal couple ended when they went looking for brief "new sensations."

It is said that, in the end, "the love you bring is the love you take," and that is usually true. But we have tried to go beyond simple phrases and jokes.

That is why we think that you will find this small manual very useful. And though it is hardly worth mentioning, we insist, once again, on the value and importance of the most seductive and powerful aphrodisiac. Without that great aphrodisiac . . . everything else is sterile and nothing can be done . . . Good luck!

Arguments

In Northern Europe we have had a saying for centuries, and with all its variants, it retains a great deal of truth and wisdom: "**Arguments kill love**." Sometimes men are content with very little. Like all people, they like to be paid attention to. I have met sex workers whose clients pay to just talk.

Since this is about having fun, we are not going to list topics of conversation. When it comes to arguing, finding issues is rather easy. Plays, films, TV series, and life itself keep us constantly updated.

However remember that arguments are not the same as a "lovers' quarrel." The two should never be confused: even in the famous *Kama Sutra*, the latter is considered a good sign in the best of relationships.

It is easy for there to be ongoing fights and arguments in any long-term relationship. But try to contain them. When there are irreconcilable differences, it becomes more difficult to regain spontaneity and confidence in bed.

Sex for Busy
People

The "Quickie": A Dilemma?

When I wrote this book, not so long ago, we still did not have millions of websites with sexual content. The unusual presence of all kinds of sex, under special classifications, deviations, and qualities, makes you wonder. I'm gathering together some of those reflections for my next book; so for now I will mention briefly a current topic, which is **quick sex**.

The so-called "quickie" is on the opposite spectrum of this book, but it seems to be a growing practice, especially among the young. It is even said that "life is too short to practice tantric sex" (and also many couples feel somewhat odd or "insincere" repeating the exotic mantras of any of the tantric rituals, but that is another issue). We will look into these matters, as I say, in the future.

Here are some erotic and sexual tricks, grouped into three categories according to duration of **time**: the first is about five to eight minutes, the second is between ten and fifteen minutes, and finally the third is for those who have about half an hour. The fun thing about these techniques or tricks, categorized as suggestions for you (♀), for him (♂), or for both, is that they do not necessarily have to be done as "quickies." Many of them are very interesting **warm-ups** for other sexual games.

At first I thought mostly about young people: the ease with which they have access to sex often conceals many of its nuances. But as I kept writing, I realized that they could be used by everyone, so get ready because what follows is pure adrenaline . . .

Five to Eight Minutes

♂ **Little things in the kitchen.** The in-laws are coming over to eat, the kids are cleaning up their rooms, and you are in the kitchen about to boil some eggs. Remember how your partner's erection gets you seething with passion. It's time to act! These places are perfect for when you do not have a lot of time but you do not want to sit down to eat without first satisfying your lover.

He wants to help; he is not a very good cook, but his penis takes less time to get hard and ejaculate than he takes brushing his teeth. And that's great for oral sex. He gets immediate pleasure, and you do not run the risk of suffering any muscle spasms.

Kneel before him; place the palms of your hands on either side of his flaccid member and move them up and down. Pretend you're trying to light a fire, because that's just what you're doing.

After about a minute, put his erect penis in your mouth. Use your tongue to stimulate the tip of the penis. Hold his testicles by cupping your left hand, and use your right thumb to massage the back of his penis. Increase the rhythm at which you massage his testicles, moving your hand beneath them to massage the perineum. Make sure that his penis is deep inside your mouth. Many people often groan with satisfaction at that moment. Increase the speed and pressure. Soon you will have this fire going, besides the one on the stove.

♀ **Commercial break.** You're watching your favorite TV show. Then come the ads and it is time to make your man happy on the sofa. First tell him to undress from the waist down and sit on one side of the sofa. You'll also undress from the waist down, and as soon as the ads start, get to it.

With him stretched on the sofa, sit on him so that your clitoris is in front of his lips. Meanwhile, your mouth will hover over his penis. You have about three and a half minutes for a 69, just long enough to avoid a neck injury. Sit back down once the ads are over.

No matter how turned on you both may be. After all, there will be another break after just a few minutes and you can go on playing this game.

If you follow through with this, you will each orgasm at the peak of the show.

♀♂ **Stairway to heaven.** If you are different heights, it will be difficult for you to have sex standing up. But a quickie on the stairs will give you that advantage you need. Now there are many houses with stairs, and I also know of some offices where if the stairwell could only talk . . . go to that staircase that nobody uses, even better if it is on a top floor.

First position: If you are shorter than your man, go up one or two steps and put one leg over the railing so you both can balance. If he is shorter, he can go up one or two steps above you. Tilt your pelvis slightly so that your vagina is facing forward.

Second position: Uncover your butt and lean slightly back, inviting him to enter you. You can lean over the railing.

Clothing: It is better for you to wear a dress or a skirt, and for him to have a coat. So that if someone were to come up or down the stairs, you can stop immediately, and avoid giggling and blushing.

♀ **Vroom vroom.** Foreplay while one of you is driving is always a bad idea. But if you do not mind getting a little late to a party, he would love to get a *massage* on his penis once you are parked. If it is nighttime, the location does not matter. But if it is daytime, go to an underground parking garage.

Then take his penis in your hands. Caress it from the tip to the base. When you get down to the base, move your hands up in reverse. Press firmly at a steady pace.

For a change of pace, open the palm of your hand and stimulate the tip, first in one direction and then another.

If you want to experience a different and delicious feeling, use a latex glove with lubricant or hand cream. Even if you are running late, the two of you will feel more relaxed when you finally get to the party. And you can always blame it on traffic.

Most cars are usually not very comfortable, but many people find it stimulating to have sex when in theory "it is not possible."

♀ **Sports.** Your man was born with ten fingers. And now is the time for him to use three of them. Just as a three-prong plug creates a current of electricity when it is inserted into a wall outlet, this technique is perfect, especially if you are short on time, for giving your whole body an electric shock.

His lubricated thumb should lightly touch you in circles, and then focus on your clitoral region. His index finger should play around with your labia.

While his index finger begins to penetrate you, invited by your natural moisture, his ring finger should approach the anal area, an equally sensitive region with nerve endings. His three fingers must cover each of these three bases, and stimulate them with intensity.

Since he is only using one hand, he could also caress, lick, or stimulate the rest of your body at the same time.

Because he is giving special attention to multiple areas of your body, your orgasm will be extremely pleasurable.

♀ **At the movies.** Movie theaters are typical places to go on a first date or a night to get away from the kids. Try to make that night special by wearing the right lingerie.

When the lights go down, no one will wonder what you are up to. Caress each other with your hands. Encourage him to explore your body so he can discover your secret and get you wet.

The good thing about movie theaters is that there is not much else to do, apart from watching the screen. And if you play it well and manage to sit in the back of the theater, you might even get to orgasm.

Another tip, if you know that you are going to the movies: do not wear any underwear. In addition, you will find other uses for ice in your drinks, such as touching your private parts before the ice and your partner get a chance to melt.

♀ **More sex in the kitchen.** Sometimes you only see each other when you get home and when you leave home: in the kitchen in the morning and evening. So why not make of it the ideal place for a quickie?

Nobody expects a five course meal, and there is no time to experiment with new foods, or wash dishes. So this will have to be something more like fast—but no less appetizing—Italian food that can be had on the kitchen counter.

Try to wear sexy stockings or garters to start things off. Then lift up your skirt to show him that you are not wearing panties. When his erect penis pounds you for about thirty times, you will come to a boil . . .

If you have a stool in the kitchen or a washing machine, get on top of it, open your legs, look at your man seductively, and enjoy.

♀ **Pearl necklace.** This is a favorite among many men who crave variety but do not always have enough time. Massage his penis between your breasts until he comes and adorns your neck with the proof of impetuous passion and satiated desire.

Kneel before him as he leans toward you. Basically, you want to stimulate his penis with your breasts. If they are large, use both hands to bring them together and create the necessary friction with his penis. If you have small breasts, use one hand to push them together and the other hand to stimulate his penis between your breasts.

This position is ideal after exercising when you're both drenched in sweat. And you will also have towels ready to dry off your pearl necklace.

♀ **Nocturnal serenade.** Years ago, vibrators were more popular among whites and Nordic people, but today erotic or sexual toys are reaching every corner of the planet. Do not worry about bringing a vibrator into your sexual routine, especially if it is one of those nights when one of you is feeling exhausted but the other partner wants to play.

In short, remember that there are three basic types of vibrators: to stimulate the clitoris, to stimulate the G-spot, and others offering different combinations.

To find out what she likes, ask if you can watch her using a vibrator. If she gives you the go ahead, ask if you can help her use it. She can place her hands on yours and show you what she likes.

Once you are past the initial phase, you should think of a vibrator as an add-on to your sexual arsenal. Since it can continue working for you even after you have an orgasm, you can always use it to finish the job you started.

Sometimes it will be useful during foreplay to excite your lover before penetrating her. Remove the vibrator and finish things on your own, at least at first. This will remind you that the vibrator is just a fun tool, not an essential object for your relationship. Do not ever forget it!

♀ **Down and up.** Going down an elevator gives you a good opportunity for him to lower his pants. Glass elevators are not a good idea, unless you like that kind of attention. But during off peak hours, you can have sex in an elevator stopped between floors.

If you're ready for it, you will have already taken off your underwear, or worn some type that can be easily removed. Do not be afraid to give precise instructions. Suggest that he do alternate movements with his tongue.

His tongue should be flat and then pointed. Encourage him to use all of his face and to sink into you. Have him insert two fingers in your vagina while he licks your clitoris. A gentle suction always offers an interesting sensation.

Moan a little bit to let him know how much you like it. When you are done and get to the lobby, get on your knees, and tell him it's time to get up to the top floor.

♀ **Kiss me slowly.** Remember those passionate make-out sessions from your first date that made your knees weak? When you stop making out, you could be doing away with passion. So it is important for you to bring back this erotic but underrated activity.

Try to turn your goodnight kiss into something really memorable. Don't you want to get at least a little wet?

Any kiss can be unforgettable and make your "knees wobbly" if you first think of the word "seduction." If you keep that in mind, your mouth will instinctively give the most seductive kisses you've ever imagined.

Secondly, imagine that you are face to face. Play with his tongue slowly and sensually, sucking on it gently, moving your mouth up and down, and use the tip of your tongue.

Explore the roof of his mouth, which is a highly sensitive place. If your guy is not a born kisser, help him get better at it. Ask him to kiss the tip of your tongue as though it were your clitoris.

About Fifteen Minutes

♀ **Frantic tantra.** A tantric *quickie* is an oxymoron, but even regular practitioners will agree that it can sexually stimulate all day, turning on your inner fire and your inner energy. Tantric sex positions tend to be somewhat complicated and require a flexible body, trained with yoga (I recommend the book *El Arte del Tantra*, which explains the positions very clearly and how everything works). But here's an idea:

The technique of "kneeling before the doors of pleasure" works well if at first your lover's penis is not erect because you'll spare yourself a lot of wrist movements. To do this, kneel and stroke him while he is standing. After, he should stay on top and penetrate you before his penis is fully erect.

Once inside you, he should lift your legs up onto his shoulders and get on his knees. Since your legs are supported on him, his hands are free.

If you both like how it feels, he can insert one or two fingers inside you and massage your G-spot. His fingers along with his penis stimulate one of your "sacred points." It's a nice position that saves time and marks the beginning of your joint yoga practice.

In the time it takes you to shower or water the plants, you and your partner can rekindle that electric feeling that brought you together. Create these kind of situations to continue that important task you gave yourself some time ago: make your partner blush from time to time.

♀♂ **Slap and tickle.** Man, woman. Night, day. A kiss, a whip. Opposites attract, and they become each other's object of desire. How is it possible that spanking can provoke sexual pleasure? Everything is a matter of endorphins.

Interestingly, when you do not have much time to devote to pleasure, some pain can bring you to an orgasm. But you must always start with a tickle.

Feathers are ideal for this, but any light and soft object can tickle: flower petals, a silk scarf, a toothbrush, a baby brush. Tickle for five minutes. Then switch the feathers for a hand, and spank each buttock lightly and then start increasing the intensity.

Spanking (of course, it has nothing to do with domestic violence, which is unfortunately too prevalent today) should last about five minutes, which leaves you five minutes for sex.

What did you say you'd make for dinner?

♀ Is there anyone sitting here? Chairs are a turn-on.
Along with a fireman's pole, they are often must-haves at any strip club. To turn him on, start with a high-backed chair with no arm rests. Sit astride your man, kiss him, and get close until your breasts are in front of his mouth. Kneel and suck on his penis.

If you have a swivel chair, the pleasure can also be yours. Sit with no underwear on, open your legs and ask him to kneel at your feet. His mission is to slowly move the chair back and forth as his tongue goes over your clitoris.

♀ Cunnilingus during your coffee break. Many women
need at least about eight minutes to orgasm. Which means you must combine two of the greatest pleasures of life: coffee and cunnilingus during a fifteen-minute break at mid-morning or mid-afternoon. Kindly take control of your man, and say, "I love it when . . . " instead of saying "I do not like it when . . . "

Tip: Ask him to kiss you from your stomach to your thighs, from your lips to the perineum (anywhere but on your clitoris). He should start licking you gently or slowly. Tell him that, as much as you groan and moan, he should take it slow. He should also alternate the intensity of his touch.

Another tip: Ask him to use his tongue to trace each letter of the alphabet on your clitoris. The hotter you get, the cooler your coffee gets . . .

♀ Under the coat. Seduction by surprise. This is a classic
move in Hollywood movies because it almost always works and it never ceases being a fun sex game. When you get

ready for a night on the town, or you agreed to meet somewhere for a night out, wear nothing but a long coat. Do not hint at your outfit being something out of the ordinary. If you behave naturally, nobody will know that there is nothing under your coat.

Grab a fresh bottle of champagne and tell your lover that before leaving you want to celebrate with a toast. It does not have to be a big celebration. Before serving the drink, take off your coat to reveal your sexy body . . . and surprise! (you can stay there or move on to the bedroom).

♀ **The alarm clock.** If you two are always busy and your schedules are completely different, take advantage of the morning (some men prefer it because at night they are usually very tired and can't help but yawn). Morning sex is great because that's when our hormonal flow is at its highest levels. That is why your guy's penis is usually erect at that time. Our bodies are also more relaxed after sleep and, therefore, more receptive.

Set the alarm clock to go off fifteen minutes earlier than usual. Do not tell him that you did it: some evil *angel* who will brighten his day (you) is going to show up.

The first thing he should know about your plan is that upon awakening he will find his penis hardening inside your mouth. Actually, there is no better way to wake up, so set up another day when he can wake you.

Slowly, ride him until the alarm goes off. If there is someone else in the house, let them think that you are still asleep. The two of you will have a special reason to glow throughout the day.

♀ **Heavenly games.** When we are extremely busy, we tend to skip foreplay and rush to intercourse. But, have you forgotten the exquisite pleasure of kissing (making out, rather) in the park, feeling each other up at parties, and fondling each other on the couch? Spend a little less time on penetration and at least a quarter of an hour to get back to basics.

Your hormones may not be vibrating energy right now, but your technique has really improved. Breast/nipple orgasm is common among women. Ask him to caress you in circles on your chest until his ring finger and thumb end up rubbing your hard nipples.

Then have him do the same with his tongue.

Find out if there is a direct connection between his nipples and his penis. As you start to get aroused, use ice cubes to relax each other, give each other chills, and make your nipples harden. If you kneel in front of each other, you can pleasure each other.

♀♂ **A good party.** The party is great, and the hosts are happy to see you. After a few drinks, you think to yourself how lucky you are to have a lover like your partner. If this is the first time you are at that house, ask the host to show it to you, so you can find a hidden corner. If you need an excuse, say you are going to get more drinks.

Never use the bathroom because someone might knock on the door to enter. Try to do it against a bedroom door to keep anyone from coming in. Or find a dark corner. Before he penetrates you, take some time to rub his penis between your labia. If you have no lubricant handy, use your saliva so you feel tender and moist.

Once you finish, do not forget to return to the party as promised: with whiskey or snacks!

♀ **His G-spot.** This technique should last a whole fifteen minutes, the time necessary for him to remember it as a luxury blowjob. First kiss him all over his body, and then in the genital area. Then hold the base of his penis very gently. Bring just the head close to your mouth and with the tip of your tongue lick the tip of his penis for a while. When of his penis is well lubricated, gently move your thumb and fore-finger along the shaft, moving slowly up and down while you are still licking the tip.

When you start to go down on his cock, imagine that your mouth is a very wet vagina. Keep him erect and let him penetrate you slowly, even imagining it is difficult for him because your mouth is still a virgin.

Start sucking his penis with a leisurely pace, hold it with your hand and mouth, and use your free hand to touch his perineum. Wet your index finger, aim it toward his anus, and then gently proceed to insert it. You will see how he loses all his senses: his G-spot is located about two and a half inches inside and it is the shortest way to his heart.

♀ **Phone sex.** Do not underestimate the power of your phone and the ability to say naughty (or nasty) things to keep your libido high and your lover happy. Tell him with clear, detailed, and specific words what you would have him do to you, and vice versa. Describe his body and all his virtues. I know it sounds trite, but describe the clothes you're wearing and be sure to wear something very sexy. Give your man something he can imagine and then move on to sexual acts. Do not rush. Speak slowly and listen to your gasps. Pauses will help the other person imagine the rest.

One famous telephone technique is suspense. Call when you know that the other person cannot answer, and offer graphic details about what you would have them do now, tomorrow, or next week. Do not hold back if you get voice-mail or an answering machine. This way he will know to return your call right away.

♀ **Come in, please.** You're pretty wet by the desire your lover awakened in you throughout the night. But once you get home, you go out for a walk with the dog, make sure that the kids are asleep and, as you wipe off your makeup, you realize that the desire is gone. So avoid any domestic distractions and promise your lover that unless there is a babysitter at your house, you will fuck as soon as you walk through the door.

Shortly before getting home, tell your partner what you plan to do with him or her. Get them talking. In doing so, you will find out what your lover wants that night, avoiding frustrations. Make the most of this initial game, be sure to give a fabulous French kiss before continuing with your domestic activities.

♀♂ **The back seat.** Instead of arriving five minutes late to a party, try to get there fifteen minutes early. Unless you want to challenge public decency and have someone notify the authorities, stop the car in a relatively secluded place.

On your way there, if he is the one driving you can take off your panties, put your legs on the dashboard, and masturbate gently. You can also tell your partner what you are experiencing when your fingers caress your clitoris and vagina, which should make him turn off the sports radio.

Once in the parking lot, he should sit in the back seat. Get in front of him, straddling his lap, and hold on to the front seat as you move back and forth. This position allows you to control the depth, speed, and duration of the game.

♀ **Freshly squeezed juice.** Surprise him with *breakfast* in bed. Grab an orange, or other piece of ripe fruit, and cut into a piece smaller than his penis (this technique works best at room temperature). You can pierce the fruit from side to side, leaving only the skin.

Place it on the tip of his penis and begin to squeeze it. If for example your man likes mangos, cut a ripe mango in half, take out the pit, and eat the flesh with a spoon. Leave a thin layer of mango pulp on his skin, and then masturbate with it.

The feeling is fantastic and his penis also acquires a sweet flavor. You will get messy, so you'd better have a towel ready to dry off the juice. What a special way to start the day, right?

♀ **Just a little.** There's something deliciously decadent about doing inappropriate things at the workplace. Take action and put on a pair of stockings and a skirt, bring a vibrator in your purse, and head to his office once all other employees have gone home. Let him know you'll come to pick him up with something to eat and do not stay more than fifteen minutes.

Sit on his desk and tell him to remain seated in his chair in front of you. Slowly open your legs so he can see your stockings, then take out your vibrator. Tell him you would like to offer him a snack before the main course, which is waiting at home.

Push forward slightly so that your vagina is at the edge of the desk, and ask him to lick your clitoris as he penetrates you with the vibrator. Once you come—combining the vibrator with the tongue is usually delicious, and it will not take you too long—turn around and bare your butt provocatively and invitingly. Let him penetrate you for a few thrusts, but not too many. Then turn away, put your toy back in the purse, and go home to wait for him because he will be there right away.

♀ **Not a whisker.** Busy couples combine personal care and foreplay because nothing is more arousing than two clean bodies rubbing together. Another advantage of having no pubic hair is that it does not get in the way during oral sex.

Go to a good professional to remove all your pubic hair: the area will be left feeling very soft and it will last longer. If you do it yourself, try shaving with an electric razor; it is safer and less painful, but it will likely feel itchy when the hair begins to grow.

♀ **Oral ice cream.** Use ice cream to improve your oral skills and your partner's. Do not spread it on his penis, just get a cone, bite off the bottom, and place it over his still flaccid penis. Now add the ice cream and start licking it until your man's penis is so hard that it breaks the cone. Or you can hold ice cubes in your mouth.

He can explore around your vaginal lips and stimulate the clitoris with the tip of his cold tongue. You will get such a surprising feeling that it will turn you on even more.

After trying this technique several times, try filling your mouth with tea or chocolate (hot without burning, of course). He won't know what's going on when the temperature goes from arctic to tropical. In any case, this exercise will have you both moaning with pleasure in no time.

♂ **Dark rain.** Shower together at night or in the dark. Being in the dark will stimulate your sense of touch. Once you get in the shower, have him wash your body slowly and sensually. He can start lathering you from behind, your back, back of your hips, calves, even your feet. And as he kneels, turn around so he can lather you starting at the bottom, up to your belly, until reaching your breasts.

Do not let him forget your arms, neck and, of course, he should lather his hand to properly wash your vagina.

If he can handle it, he can lift you up to get your legs to wrap around his waist, and he can start to penetrate you. Let the water soak your body while you make love.

If you want to howl with excitement, he can stretch over the tub and you can ride him. Is there anything better than this?

♀ **Get up and get going.** Are you sick of having to clean your house? Are you tired of housework? Any time you are standing upright is great for a quickie. Put away the vacuum cleaner and get to work!

If your man is a little taller than you, or it is the other way around, get on a stepping stool or a phone book. Let him bend his knees a little bit so he can penetrate you more easily and pick you up. If you are a yogi or an athlete, lean on one leg and put the other one around him. You may not have much freedom of movement, but he can do a circling motion as he penetrates you. You can both lean against a wall. In that case, put your arms around his neck as he lifts you up from your hips or under your butt. You just have to wrap your legs around his hips.

♀ **Massage.** Sometimes one of you wants to have sex but the other does not. What is the fastest way to turn on your partner? Offer him a quick massage. Put on his favorite song or sensual music to help him relax. Pour a generous amount of massage oil in the palm of your hand and rub your hands together. With warm hands, gently caress his back, chest, arms, and hands. Once he is feeling relaxed, you can start with the sexy part of the massage.

He can do the same for you and then gently massage your vulva, followed by stimulation of the clitoris, and then do some internal and clitoral stimulation at the same time.

He can also stimulate your G-spot with his index and ring finger. Then bend his fingers together rhythmically inside the vagina (indicating "come here").

To massage his genitals you slow down the amount of stimulation until you stop or change course before getting to the point of no return.

First alternate your caresses and then concentrate on one or two when the end is near. If your lover has an orgasm without ejaculating, extend his erection, so that afterward his orgasm will be even more intense.

♀ **Get undressed.** He can first choose a song you like and that he can move to. If he is dancing for you, choose a song that has some meaning. Then, he should plan that last step when he makes himself known and wears his sexiest clothes to surprise you.

You get to sit down as he turns off the lights, lighting only a few candles for you to enjoy the show. He can put on music and get on stage, then move sensually and start to undress, showing off his back and taking off his shirt. He can give you a few lap dances so you can enjoy his body from all possible angles. You are allowed to smell but not touch him. He has to take off all his clothes and toss them to you.

When he gets down to his last clothing item, he will move even more slowly, taking off his underwear until it is down at his ankles. He can flex his arms to draw attention away from his belly. Bring his hands to his knees and shake his ass. Dancing seductively. He should take off his socks and shoes gently. If he has done it well, before the show is over you too should be undressed.

♀♂ **Knots.** Quick sex implies speeding up the sexual game. After talking about some of your partner's fantasies, you can explore one that is more common than it seems: bondage.

If you feel comfortable and fully trust your partner, ask him if he would want to be tied up gently (you should never just surprise him with something like this). Once you have permission, first try tying his hands. Something as simple as a kiss on the cheek tastes different when one of you is tied.

Then try to tie his feet (also softly) to limit his movement. This feeling of helplessness adds excitement and erotic experimentation. Remember that you should never tie him up too tightly so that his blood can continue flowing normally.

You can use silk ties or something similar, or a silk scarf, but always listen to your partner without forcing any physical bondage. Some people admit to getting aroused when they are gently tied with extreme care.

Thirty Minutes

♀♂ **Three positions.** You know, your sex life can always be the same, or it can always be a little different. Stop thinking "we are always doing the same thing," and try alternating three different positions in a single session. Half an hour goes a long way for sexual positions. Just warn your man that he will have to do a little more work.

Start with a "usual" position you already know and like, but after ten minutes switch to a new one. After another ten minutes, move on to another one. The following combinations work well and do not require a lot of effort:

Doggy style, stretched forward, and then lopsided: Begin on all fours. He penetrates you from behind. Then both of you lean forward and stretch on the bed, but he stays on top of you. To get more stimulus, slide your hand between your legs and stimulate your clitoris. And finally, turn sideways. This allows you to stimulate each other mutually and have an orgasm.

Missionary position, then neck and shoulders: He should be on top of you, but after ten minutes lift your legs over his neck. It will be much easier if he lifts your legs and holds them.

Finally, place your hands at the base of your hip to lift, so that the full weight of your body rests on your shoulders. This allows for a really deep penetration (and is ideal if your guy is not well endowed).

Cowgirl position, then sideways: Ride him and look into his eyes. After ten minutes, stretch over him so that your clitoris is in close contact with his pubic bone while he continues to penetrate you. Then turn on your sides and finish what you started!

♀♂ **Come again.** Like the idea of having orgasms so intense that they leave you shaking? Why have just one orgasm if you can have two? Take turns so that the two of you can repeat your orgasms, and those will have been thirty minutes well spent.

♂ **Men:** Give her a clitoral orgasm followed by a G-spot orgasm. The easiest way to make her come is by stimulating the clitoris through oral sex. Women usually prefer lighter pressure than men, so be discreet when licking, moving your tongue over her labia and thighs, and on the clitoris.

Once she comes, stop touching the clitoris because it is very sensitive. Slide one or two fingers in her vagina and find the G-spot (about 2 or 3 inches inside the upper wall of the vagina). You'll notice that it begins to swell. Press firmly upwards and with a little luck, it will swell even more. Press harder and see how she comes and *squirts* at the same time.

♀ **Women:** Forget about any prejudices and go for a good old fashioned prostate orgasm. Start by covering a finger with lubricant, then gently touch him around the anus. Let him know what is going on, otherwise his anus will contract, and you do not want that. As he relaxes, firmly place your finger on the contour of his anus to find the opening.

Insert your finger slowly until you feel his prostate (a hazelnut-shaped bulb located about six or seven centimeters inside the anus) and then press firmly. As you press down on it, you will feel it swelling. He will begin to feel tingling and intense sensations all over his body. He may ejaculate, but in this case it would not be due to an orgasm.

With a little luck, he will not ejaculate until you stop and return to your usual ways of making him come. Try a blowjob (after washing your hands) or manual stimulation of the penis.

He will not be able to hide his smile for weeks!

♀ **Punishment and reward.** You think tying someone is the finest form of slavery? Think again. Tonight you are going to dominate your man without any tools. I can guarantee that it is much more intense to restrict his movements only using your mind. And you will have to boss him around, which is not bad: order him to get on the bed and tell him that you will let him know what positions you want. (Reassure him that you are not going to ask him to wash a pile of dirty dishes.)

When he is in a position you like, he will not be allowed to move, no matter what you do. You can threaten him with a whip if he does not do exactly as you order. Then open his legs and place his hands behind his head.

Now start to tickle him unmercifully. Kneel on him, facing his feet. Starting at his feet, kiss him all over. Use your tongue on his toes and instep. If he gets ticklish, massage his feet to desensitize them a bit. Start at his ankles (about an inch outside of his ankle, there is a very erotic acupressure point), legs, inner thighs, and penis. Stop there for a moment before continuing to the stomach, chest, nipples, neck, ears, and lips. Surely, by then he will be desperate to penetrate you, so stop him from moving by placing his hands over his head while you kiss him.

Then move slowly to his genitals and wrap it up with hot oral sex. If you feel really stingy, masturbate in front of him. Tell him if he behaves, you will make sure he comes too, but he must remain completely still with his hands where you can see them.

You'll have intense orgasms, because the best sex always begins in the mind.

♀♂ **Synchronicity.** Try oriental-style sex, in which you use sensual and sensory elements. If you start practicing it with your partner, he will think you're the most sensual lover in the world.

In addition, you will not need to make love for seven hours; it is possible to live certain tantric experiences in thirty minutes. It is important to remember that tantra has more to do with connection through sex, but orgasms can be so intense that you just end up forming a very deep connection with the other person.

Begin by playing soothing music, lighting candles, and getting undressed. Now sit in front of your partner and look into his eyes. You may want to start giggling. If so, laugh, relax, and enjoy these moments of intimacy. After five minutes, bring your lips together and take turns feeling each other's breath. Synchronize your breathing for greater intensity, but stop if either of you gets dizzy.

After five minutes, touch each other's palms without looking away. Feel the warmth of your skin and the energy flowing between you two. Do this for five minutes and then massage your chakras.

Remember that there are seven chakras. The root chakra is located between your anus and genitals (your perineum). Then comes the orange chakra located at the center of your abdomen. Go up and you will find the solar plexus chakra, then the heart and neck. Then comes the brow/third eye chakra (located in the center of your forehead between the eyes), and finally the crown chakra, at the top of your head.

To massage your chakras, use your fingers and go from one chakra to the next, starting from the first to the last. Make it last ten minutes, or more time if you have it. When you are done, the two of you will feel so connected and excited that the last five minutes for this massage can be used for very intense sex.

Other Tricks to Fuel Your Fire

♀♂ **In a moment.** One way to ensure that your partner reaches an orgasm faster is to accelerate the intensity of your touch during lovemaking. Try slight scratches, bites, or moderate grips.

This should not hurt, of course, but should be strong enough to awaken his senses. Start very gently and then increase pressure gradually. On a scale of one to ten, where one would be an almost imperceptible caress and ten would be painful contact, do not go past a five.

Gently biting or pinching the nipples in males and females usually produces a warm feeling in our sexual organs and activates our bodily fluids. A key part of this shortcut is the surprise factor, so it is important not to overdo it (do not hurt your partner!).

If you're about to come and see that your partner is not there yet, increase your intensity; try pinching or biting a little harder.

♀ **Good vibrations.** A vibrator is the fastest way to go from "Oh, no" to "Oh, please, yes, yes!" But you have to know how to use it. It is not enough to simply press it against your clitoris and expect instant gratification. Your clitoris is delicate and if you misuse it you will only end up damaging your nerve endings and it will take you hours to get aroused. It is best to start outside your pleasure center.

Turn your vibrator to the lowest setting and start pressing it against the contours of your clitoris. After a minute, move it until it touches the side of the clitoris. Mmmm . . . it feels good, right? Now turn up the speed a little bit and press it so that the tip of the device moves up and down along your clitoris. Press it hard against you and feel as though you are about to explode, turn it to full speed. Bam! You finish and your batteries did not die.

♀ **Panties.** What kind of panties should you wear for a fit of passion? The kind with ties at the sides. Tie them with soft loop and they will fall to the ground with his touch. Otherwise, try thongs, which are not only exciting but also give easy access to the vagina and are ideal for a meeting with a sex buddy.

If you wear panties and stockings with garters you can take them off by doing a striptease that your partner will enjoy. Or wear only discreet panties that will not get in the way.

When you go out, tell him you forgot to wear panties and invite him to touch you. If you've done your homework, he will not need an invitation to join your party.

♀ **Lubricant.** You would never make an egg salad sandwich without mayonnaise, right? Vegetables without dressing are very bland. How would a car run without gasoline? Lubricants always make things better and sex is no exception.

For women, one of the drawbacks of having quickies is that they have no time to get naturally lubricated. We do not always have time to get turned on slowly and sensually to the point where we are wet, although rules for good sex are not negotiable: his penis must be erect and she has to be moist.

Often, a drop of lubricant is the answer. Generally speaking, a woman is never sufficiently lubricated, so keep a lubricant in your bedroom and even carry some in your bag. There are plenty of soft lubricants for sale, even some that taste like strawberry or banana and are water soluble, just in case more lubrication is needed.

♀ **Shower.** If you never used the shower faucet for other purposes, now is your chance. There are two types of faucets for nice clean fun. With one, you can move it to get a strong water jet going. With the other, you can get a variety of massages and vibrations.

Find one that feels comfortable and make sure the water temperature is warm, not very hot. Start with moderate pressure and increase it gradually.

Try to direct water to different points: you can choose between a direct jet to your clitoris (something intensely erotic) or vibrant rain on your labia (but not inside the vagina because that could be dangerous).

Try to spray directly at your clitoris. You will feel a sensation similar to when a man licks you. However, do not focus all your attention to the area between your legs because the water jet can also delight you in other parts of your body.

♀ **Squeezes.** Some women get sexual pleasure—even an orgasm–from simply squeezing their hips. There is no secret because this action indirectly stimulates the clitoris. You can practice this discreet technique anywhere, even in public!

Are you traveling by train and you are still several hours away from your destination? Are you bored with work in the office? Now it is time to have fun. Did you ever try doing this? You can practice at home when you're lying in bed:

Cross your feet at your ankles, then with rhythmic movements, tighten your hips, fantasize, and occasionally touch your nipples if you have trouble reaching orgasm just by squeezing. Another way is to cross your legs and place an ankle over the other leg, creating pressure on the clitoris.

Some women prefer to "press against the seam" of their jeans or tights, while others love to do it with bare legs under a skirt or dress.

Experiment until you find what you like. But be careful; if you practice this technique to the point of perfecting it, you run the risk of getting turned on every time you sit down.

♀ **Multi-orgasmic.** On your next hot date, go to the toilet whenever you can and masturbate.

That will get you lubricated, and keep in mind that every time you masturbate, you send blood to your vagina, stimulating nerve endings, and increasing your chances for experiencing multiple orgasms when you make love with someone. You will have more "multiple orgasms."

Use your right index finger and thumb to cover your clitoris. Move your fingers in circles. Repeat throughout the day. Then you might have to warn your partner that you will be ready for him when you see each other.

♂ **Venus butterfly.** If you want a shortcut for her to have an orgasm, go straight to the source: the clitoris. The clitoris has thousands of nerve endings. Much like your penis, it fills with blood and becomes rigid when she is excited.

You will want to respect the fact that her clitoris is the most sensitive part of her body. Avoid licking or handling it with excessive force or without lubrication. What she needs is a constant and repetitive motion in one or both sides of her clitoris. Generally women have a favorite side, so ask her what she likes.

Find her clitoris by opening her labia and pulling on them gently. Once you find it, lick it quickly and smoothly. Do not use your teeth or a hard sucking motion when you start. Lick the wall of the clitoris so that your tongue forms a V shape. Go slowly.

Caress and gently pinch her labia. Pull them gently until she moans. Then lick and suck around her clitoris but not in it. Wait till she asks. Keep in mind that this is very intimate. The more excited she is, the more (or less) she will want you to directly stimulate her clitoris. Be sure to discuss it before you start. Remember that after an orgasm the clitoris may retract and become very sensitive to any further stimulus to the point of being painful.

Repair
Manual

It is very hard to get your heart and head together in life. Mine aren't even friendly.

(CRIMES AND MISDEMEANORS)

What to Do If . . .

This is the final part of our manual. Sometimes (more often than we think) sex does not work out well, so we have prepared a short list of "malfunctions" and ways to fix them. The disorder or abnormalities "catalog" is broad, although fortunately having to visit the doctor is becoming less frequent.

■ **Acupuncture**. It has been an essential part of traditional Chinese medicine for thousands of years. There are thought to be meridians running throughout the human body circulating vital energy, which sometimes flows insufficiently or is blocked. Energy dysfunctions can be attributed to emotional or physical shock. To balance this energy, needles are pinned on specific points of our skin, directly connecting to the affected organs. The needles have an incredible energy rebalancing power and they are pain-free. This treatment can be combined with homeopathy or other natural remedies, which are as harmless as they are effective.

■ **Affection**. Besides respect this is a basic component for good sex, whether we are in a committed relationship or with someone we just met. Affection gives us self-confidence and lessens our inhibitions for sex.

■ **Anorgasmia**. It occurs when a woman cannot reach an orgasm, even when she may feel aroused and lubricated, her genitals swell, and she experiences all kinds of erotic impulses. It is a physical impediment, since desire remains latent in women suffering from this disorder. It is the most common female sexual dysfunction. There are two types of anorgasmia: lifelong, when the woman has never experienced an orgasm; and situational, when it occurs only under certain circumstances. In this sense, popular belief, not science, differentiates an orgasm reached through clitoral stimulation rather than from vaginal intercourse. After conducting extensive studies, experts have come to agree that both types of orgasm are equally important. We must clarify that a woman who does not reach orgasm through intercourse is not necessarily suffering anorgasmia.

■ **Anxiety**. It is the body's response to any threats, both real and imaginary. The body is on alert and ready for flight or fight, as in any stressful situation. It increases blood flow in the heart and muscles, while decreasing it in areas that are not used for fight or flight responses, including the genitals. Therefore anxiety prevents blood from flowing to the penis and prevents erections. The greatest impediment for an erection is anxiety. So try not to make love if you are feeling worried or thinking about other things > Stress.

- **Aphrodisiacs**. Traditionally it is said that their powers are mysterious and debatable: neither rhino horn nor a product called "Spanish fly" have been proven effective, except in that they can cause tissue irritation. However, ginseng, or many other foods, such as celery, have a slight erotic effect.

  Others, such as royal jelly or shellfish, are simply foods that provide vitamins, minerals, and trace elements (such as zinc, for example) that have valuable revitalizing power. There is a third group of newly created products that promise sexual enjoyment, like drinks with added supplements (for instance, taurine), but its real power is less than what the ads promise. We need to make a clear distinction between these products and drugs like Viagra that is useful only in case of erectile dysfunction under medical supervision. It is best to consult a doctor before using any of these products because some of them have significant side effects.

- **Arguments**. This topic deserves its own chapter due to how important they are to relationships and sex life. There are a lot of myths regarding arguments, and we think that the only silver lining is making up, mostly in bed. With reoccurring arguments, it is easy to lose mutual respect, but respect is essential for an emotionally and sexually healthy relationship. Just as with anxiety and stress, arguing overworks our mind with thoughts of what we said and heard, and we are left incapable of feeling sexual desire.

- **Bachelor(ette) parties**. This tradition that is so ingrained in our society does nothing to enrich the couple's life; it offers nothing good. Each partner goes out on their own with a group of people rushing to get into situations they think they will not be able to do once married. Nothing could be further from reality, and it is a deceptive practice that we should do away with.

■ **Backache**. People who suffer from pain in the back, neck, or kidneys, participate more passively during sex, for example by lying on their back and avoiding any kind of pressure. The same applies for any other kind of pain, although there are certain positions that are better for those suffering pain in the back or kidneys. If the woman is the one who feels pain, then her partner can lie on top of her, supporting his weight on his arms to avoid excessive pressure on her. If the man is the one who feels pain, he can sit in a chair with his back straight and the woman can straddle him. Another good position is with the woman kneeling forward and him standing behind her; making sure that the vagina is at the same level as the penis and that the man's back remains straight.

■ **Birth control pill**. It is very commonly used by women. Its creation in the sixties was a real revolution for most women, as it meant that they could freely decide whether to be mothers or not. It also led to changes in sexual behavior. Birth control pills are becoming more sophisticated each day, although they still have unwanted side effects. A trend among family planning specialists is combining more than one contraceptive method to avoid such effects. One side effect may be lower sexual desire.

■ **Breasts**. Breasts are not only intended for feeding children after birth. Remember that this is an erogenous zone that is an active part of female sexuality and sexually appealing for many men. If you lose sensitivity in your breasts, go see a specialist. Clamps and other devices meant to increase blood flow to this area may eventually become painful and have unwanted effects.

■ **Condoms**. We have seen an increase in sexually transmitted diseases, so it is not surprising that health authorities, or any specialists in any forum, advocate condom use as much or more as a tool for disease prevention as for birth control. Why are so many men bothered by having to wear condoms then? It could be linked to the desire for a more *intense* sexual relationship, wanting to experience a mutual flow of energies that turns the sexual act into what the French call "a little death." This can facilitate, if the situation allows, a view into the threshold of infinity, and receiving energy that is released in female vaginal secretions.

■ **Contraceptives**. They help prevent unwanted pregnancies or regulate menstrual cycles in women. Beyond oral contraceptives (pills), there are two kinds of birth control: mechanical, such as a condom, diaphragm, cervical cap, or sponge, which create a physical barrier between sperm and eggs; and chemical contraceptives that destroy sperm.

■ **Creativity**. Sexual creativity is very directly related to eroticism and helps us cope with routine in a long-term relationship. Being creative in our relationships will help us feel more excited about our sex life, which is often hampered through monotony. Without necessarily doing anything "eccentric," we can use our imagination and try new experiences that will enrich our relationship. Naturally, we should be creative in all aspects of our lives; in fact, there are self-help courses on how to be more creative.

■ **Delayed ejaculation**. Those who suffer from this disorder can stay erect during sexual intercourse without any problems, but often have difficulty ejaculating. The problem can be mild and overcome by lengthening the amount of time that the penis is stimulated; but it worsens when this method does not work. Some men are unable to ejaculate inside a vagina, but have no trouble ejaculating when they are stimulated orally or by hand. This type of case can worsen if he is able to ejaculate by masturbating.

Until just a few years ago, delayed ejaculation was less common than premature ejaculation. This is due to changes in our sexual mores and generally false beliefs that women take longer to orgasm than men. For this reason, to catch up to women, men have sharply tried slowing down and interrupting their natural responses.

■ **Depression**. When we are depressed, we tend to lose interest in sex. Weighed down by problems, depressed people need to work on themselves as individuals before starting a relationship. Keep in mind that depression can impact the functioning of the body and change the endocrine system affecting our libido. It can decrease androgen levels and neurotransmitters such as *serotonin* (which decreases sexual activity) and *norepinephrine* (which increases it). Both play an important role in our emotional health. It is important to rule out any type of depression or emotional stress before starting sexual therapy.

■ **Dirty sex**. The boundary between what we consider dirty, or not, is in our minds. Tradition, culture, and religion taught us that sex is sinful, but now that we know that it is not, what do we do about some behaviors that are abhorrent to some but not to others? We look for "respect" as we keep in mind that the best guarantee for enjoying sex is the complicity between two people and taking responsibility for what we do.

■ **Disaffection**. If love is the best aphrodisiac, indifference can completely cancel out any sexual desire. Rarely do we worry about anyone experiencing estrangement, but it can cause suffering with the same intensity but in different ways. If your partner makes you feel insignificant, then the desire to make love with him disappears. Many men and women, afraid to confront their estranged partner, have sex with them without having anything real to offer and suffer in silence. There are several reasons for disaffection in a relationship: infidelity, routine, no attraction, and, very commonly, focusing on a third person that makes us undervalue our current partner.

■ **Drugs and stimulants**. We touched on this before: science tells us that alcohol, coffee, and tobacco hinder sex. But there are other substances that can act as aphrodisiacs (such as yohimbe), stimulants (such as coca leaf), or relaxants (hemp, for example). Their effects vary because they have a high psychological influence. As we said throughout this book, we do not recommend using drugs or designer drugs. To enjoy many years of a happy sex life, it is better to rely on more natural elements. As for pharmaceuticals, note that they can interfere with nerves or nerve impulses that control blood vessels. For example, drugs for treating ulcers or gastrointestinal disorders, antidepressants, antihistamines, blood pressure medications, or diuretics. The results worsen if taken in combination or with alcohol.

■ **Endocrine glands**. The endocrine system includes the pituitary gland found in the skull and is responsible for secreting hormones. These, in turn, stimulate other glands such as the testes or ovaries to secrete androgens. Androgens are also hormones that, much like testosterone, activate or decrease sexual functioning in the brain. Depending on how much of these hormones there is in our blood, sexual desire will increase or disappear. Therefore, changes to the normal functioning of the endocrine glands may cause sexual disorders or dysfunctions.

■ **Fantasies**. A sensual atmosphere is necessary for lovemaking to be a pleasant experience. That is why fantasizing is an important part of any erotic relationship, and much like creativity, fulfilling a sexual fantasy helps to break routine and monotony.

Be in tune with your partner's desires and fantasies. Wearing erotic clothing or decorating a room should be for your mutual enjoyment. As we mentioned earlier on quirks, fantasy depends on mutual respect and the pursuit of sexual pleasure for both. Certain unfulfillable fantasies can be substituted to avoid frustration of wanting something and not getting it.

■ **Flirting**. It is not only a physical seduction. Silly games and baby talk give us a sense of helplessness and need for affection, often tied to pranks and fun shenanigans.

■ **Forbidden**. "What is forbidden is desired." "Is it forbidden to forbid?" Social changes and the new millennium bring a new system of values in a world increasingly populated by "lonely crowds." Every time something appears to be forbidden to us, we ourselves can form emotional barriers that prevent us from cautiously and responsibly enjoying sex as a natural part of life.

■ **Frigidity**. In this case, at the physiological level, the vagina does not lubricate, and psychologically, women do not feel any erotic impulses. Sexual ability becomes inhibited more or less, depending on the severity of the disorder. The woman does not experience any pleasure and may feel aversion to sex.

She may agree to have sex when she feels that it is her *duty* and may get some pleasure from being useful to her man, or she may avoid it altogether. Despite not feeling sexual impulses, some women can orgasm when properly stimulated, usually in the clitoris. The worst feeling a frigid woman experiences is being excluded and used by her partner, since she does not experience sex as a pleasurable act.

■ **Guilt**. The most common feelings of guilt in relation to sex are a result of religious education, which has always associated sexual pleasure with sin. Our cultural education also impacts our inhibitions when it comes to viewing sex as a natural part of life. Society is no longer as influenced by religion or weighed down by tradition and culture, but other things tend to affect us individually and make us feel guilty for being unable or not ready to meet our partner's expectations for a satisfying sex life. In this sense, friends' comments, though innocent, can be very harmful.

■ **Impotence**. It is one of the most frustrating physical changes for a man. In short, it is a lack of blood flow to the penis, preventing it from staying erect long enough for intercourse. When this anomaly is reoccurring, it is *generalized* impotence, whereas situational impotence may occur at a particular time, if he is under stress or pressure, or drank too much alcohol, or in an unexpected situation. The most curious case would be a man who suffers from selective impotence; that is to say, his penis gets erect long enough to make love with certain women but not with others. Impotence can be a warning sign for other diseases, such as diabetes.

- **Incompatibilities**. It is commonplace to hear, "Whenever he wants it, I don't." Fortunately we are not all the same: it is logical that we do not always feel sexual desire at the same time. Come to terms with this because it is essential to understanding your partner. In addition, never make the mistake of having sex just to please the other person. Another myth related to (in)compatibilities is *simultaneous orgasm*, which only rarely happens. The important thing is for you both to feel pleasure making love.

- **Loss of sexual appetite**. If, after trying these tricks and tips you feel as though there is "nothing to do," you're with an alien who vibrates at a different frequency; consider other solutions. Try living!

- **Masturbation**. The line between fondling and masturbation is sometimes wonderfully blurred, but the fact is that we Westerners have been made to feel so guilty with sermons against masturbation that we ended up on the opposite extreme.

  However, let us remember what the great sages of the East have said on this subject: "It is really important for man to avoid ejaculating at all costs." What is certain is that moderate masturbation between couples can become a way of enhancing and enriching their sex life and increasing levels of intimacy.

- **Medication**. When taking any drug, keep in mind that it can adversely affect your sex life.

  For instance, medication for gastrointestinal disorders, anxiolytics, and antihistamines interfere with nerve impulses that control blood vessels in the penis and block some nerves, which would prevent erections. Other medications, however, directly affect our mood and prevent us from feeling sexual desire.

- **Mystery**. Sometimes an aura of mystery in the relationship is very appealing. On the other hand, not being able to freely express our feelings can end the relationship. Silence creates a situation of uncertainty which can initially intrigue your partner, but if it is sustained for long, it can lead to an untenable situation that could even result in a break up. Be mysterious but in moderate doses.

- **Obligation**. Forcing someone to have sex is a violent act that should not be tolerated. In the past, women were not aware that they could refuse sex with their husbands, but today's society makes it clear that what once seemed normal is unhealthy behavior.

  Do not give in to someone else's desire if you do not want sexual intercourse. It is best to find some middle ground, where both partners feel comfortable.

- **Orgasm**. Orgasm is considered the pinnacle of all sexual relations, but there is no reason to blow it out of proportion because not getting there could lead to frustration. For both men and women, the physical state after an orgasm is complete relaxation and satisfaction, but they differ in that women can orgasm in two different ways (vaginal stimulation or clitoris) but men in only one way (through stimulation of the penis).

- **Pain**. Pain in the man's genitals, when not due to physiological reasons, is often associated with irritations or disorders resulting from promiscuity and lack of hygiene, such as venereal diseases.

When a woman feels pain in the genitals, (*dyspareunia*), during or after intercourse, it may be due to physical or psychological reasons. In the first case, it has mostly to do with vaginal or vulvar lesions, inflammation, and vaginal infections, using irritating feminine hygiene products, or due to dryness of the vagina resulting from hormonal changes. Vaginal cysts or scarring from an operation can also cause pain during intercourse. However, pain is often linked to the woman's emotional state, for example when the man is uncaring. Sexual violence or cultural or religious fears may also have some influence. Once you rule out physical reasons, try talking to a therapist to work out any emotional reasons. > Vaginismus.

■ **Phimosis**. This is a typical problem for men. It is a tightness of the foreskin that prevents its retraction over the glans of the penis. It can be painful during lovemaking, but it can be easily solved with surgery (circumcision).

■ **Physical**. Although physical appearance is very important, there are other prevalent aspects (in addition to the purely aesthetic) for attraction to exist between a man and a woman. Note that aesthetics depend on ever changing fashion and beauty standards.

For a good physical response, start by being yourself and feel satisfied with your appearance. Loving yourself, liking who you are, and pampering your body makes it easier for others to notice you. Feeling ashamed with your appearance is the greatest disservice you can do to yourself if you want to be appreciated by others. Avoid using phrases such as "I cannot stand myself," or "I would get surgically remade, if I could." These attitudes are naive or teenage nonsense.

- **Porn**. There is specific pornographic material for homo-sexuals and other groups, but the vast majority of porn magazines, movies, or videos are made with a typical male mentality (not to mention vulgar), and include numerous scenes to express submission in one way or another. In addition, there is porn depicting scenes that could hardly be considered erotic (bestiality, for example) by a large majority of people. Pornography does not contribute much to sexual liberation. It can give you some hints, but keep in mind that it generally follows a pattern of exaggeration and grossness. Like a circus, these materials claim impossible feats and insist that "the show must go on."

- **Premature ejaculation**. Some men have a difficult time controlling ejaculation, and when they reach a certain level of excitement, they tend to ejaculate quickly. Not all sexologists agree on why a man has or develops pre-mature ejaculation. For some, it has to do with the time it takes to ejaculate once intercourse begins; however, others have a direct inability to control it.

  It has nothing to do with feeling arousal or getting an erection because many men suffering from prema-ture ejaculation enjoy normal erections. Sometimes they can ejaculate during foreplay and even at the sight of a female body without any additional help. The most com-mon therapies are based on making him recognize and get used to the feeling of an approaching ejaculation, so that he can start controlling them.

- **Priapism**. Having a permanently erect penis was erro-neously considered as inexhaustible fertility and sexual pleasure. Or so they thought in ancient Greece where this notion was shaped into Priapus, their god of fertility on earth. Nothing could be further from the truth: this is a permanent and painful erectile dysfunction accompanied by an absence of sexual desire. It may be caused by some type of infection in the urethra or prostate or a neurological dysfunction. It requires urgent medical treatment.

- **Prolonging pleasure**. This is a dream goal for many couples, and why not? Increasingly we hear of certain Eastern philosophies and practices aimed at prolonging sexual pleasure. In Tantra, for example, there are men who can orgasm multiple times without ejaculating. There are also tools: rings that when placed correctly on the penis, can help him maintain an erection for longer and prolong the sexual act. Or so they say.

- **Psychology**. We insist that this book does not address issues related to conventional or academic psychology. It is a manual to help you enjoy sexuality. But psychological elements abound and don't we all tend to guard our own personal neuroses? We could say that psychology is present in many of your sexual encounters, more than you think. It is often said that "sex is in the brain"; that is, it would not kill you to look into books on humanistic psychology or self-help.

- **Quirkiness**. "I do not care about quirkiness. Sometimes he was fascinated with my pubic hair, then it was all about walking naked on all fours, then . . . " This type of comment is not surprising. Both men and women have their own fantasies, but understand that what may be very erotic and stimulating for some, others could consider uncomfortable and even annoying.

- **Sacred sex**. It is expected to become a big trend in the coming years, so remember: you are a *goddess*, and as the Taoist sage says, "In heaven and under heaven: *everything* is sacred."

- **Scents**. In addition to a pleasant environment, pay attention to your personal scent. Someone said that "love begins with perfumes and it ends when *other* smells appear . . . " So pay attention to your own breath as much as you can and accept (also as much as you can) the other person's. But from our breath all the way to our most intimate corners, we must learn to engage with our own scents and those of others. Certain private parts give off a particular smell and men and women get used to them if everything else takes place in a pleasant atmosphere.

- **Seduction**. It is "even better than power." That is why we find it important that others pay us some attention. Knowing how to seduce is an art, especially when we are with the same person for a long time and we still manage to surprise, seduce, and ultimately encourage him to make love, no matter how tired or worried we may be. To be a good seducer or seductress we do not need to be extraordinarily good looking; as we mentioned in a previous section, there are other even more powerful elements than our appearance (which we should still care about, of course).

- **Sexually transmitted diseases (STDs).** Only by practicing responsible and safe sex can we stop these diseases from spreading from individuals to the rest of society. Some STDs are difficult to detect because symptoms appear later than usual or do not last very long, and when they finally seem to disappear, the disease may still be present. Some of these infections can be cured with simple antibiotics, but others, such as AIDS or herpes, still lack a definitive treatment. It is also important to be aware that once you are infected, the disease can spread to others in an endless chain. The most common sexually transmitted diseases are gonorrhea, chlamydia, genital herpes, AIDS, and syphilis.

- **Simultaneous Orgasm** > Incompatibilities.

- **Stress**. Do not make love under stressful situations, or in a rush (give yourself at least a couple of hours, for example). As we know, our current pace of life is stressful and this tension causes relationship problems. Faced with a stressful situation, our body starts preserving energy and uses just enough energy to help us solve the problem at hand. Sex does not start in bed, but much earlier, and thinking that you can make love at any time, day or night, is not realistic. You need some preparation and your partner has to be willing, of course. Sometimes stressful situations occur when one of the partners (sometimes both) feel pressured or stressed when making love because it is not an ideal time for them.

- **Tears**. The tears of a man can have an erotic effect for some women, either because it brings out their maternal instinct or protective and nurturing feelings. Some men instinctively try to seem helpless for this purpose. The situation does not usually occur in reverse.

- **Testosterone**. It is the quintessential natural aphrodisiac. It is the only natural substance that can increase sexual desire in men due to its effect on particular points in the brain. The testicles are responsible for making it and thus setting off erection and desire. Incidentally, it is said that bald men have a more fulfilling sex life and are more vigorous; recently, it has been confirmed that one of the reasons for baldness is excess testosterone.

- **Vaginismus**. Involuntary and spasmodic contractions of the muscle that closes the entrance of the vagina when trying to insert the penis, preventing sexual intercourse. It is the least common female sexual dysfunction and sometimes occurs in anxious or phobic personalities, with fear of penetration. Moreover these women usually orgasm through clitoral stimulation since what they really fear is actual penetration.

- **Venereal** (diseases). > STD

- **Violence**. We differentiate between ill-treatment at home and sadomasochism. What passionate relationship doesn't include a little bit of S&M, at least from a psychological standpoint? In some traditional cultures there are texts on this subject, where controlled pain gives pleasure. It's not about sadomasochism, but rather about games that some couples can engage in. When it comes to sadomasochism, for many it is completely aberrant, but we'd be surprised by how many people practice it in secret. Control is essential in these cases to avoid extreme situations. There is something for everyone . . .

- **Voyeurism**. There are men who get off by watching other people engage in sexual activity. This is another reason why porn exists. In fact, most teenagers masturbate watching porn and with magazines. There are also men and women who experience more pleasure watching others in a sexual relationship rather than participating in it.

Other Books by Tina Robbins:

—201 ideas para volver loco a tu hombre en la cama
—Técnicas avanzadas para volver loco a tu hombre en la cama
—Orgasmo en 5 minutos